KIDNEY DISEASE DIET COOKBOOK FOR STAGE 3

Essential Diet Tips and Recipes for Kidney Care

Dr. Melissa R. Steven

Copyright © 2024 [Dr. Melissa R. Steven]

All rights reserved. No part of this material may be reproduced, distributed, or transmitted in any form or by any means, including photocopying, recording, or other electronic or mechanical methods, without the prior written permission of the copyright owner, except in the case of brief quotations embodied in critical reviews and certain other noncommercial uses permitted by copyright law.

INTRODUCTION

Welcome to the "Kidney Disease Diet Cookbook for Stage 3," your essential guide to managing kidney health through mindful eating. At Stage 3 kidney disease, your kidneys are moderately damaged and require special attention to prevent further decline.

Diet plays a crucial role in supporting kidney function. This cookbook focuses on balanced, kidney-friendly meals that help control protein, sodium, potassium, phosphorus, and fluid intake. By following these guidelines, you can help reduce the strain on your kidneys and improve your overall health.

Inside, you'll find practical tips for meal planning, grocery shopping, and cooking. Each chapter provides a variety of recipes for breakfast, lunch, dinner, snacks, desserts, and beverages, all tailored to meet your dietary needs. Additionally, there are special sections for vegetarian, vegan, gluten-free, and diabetic-friendly options, along with strategies for overcoming dietary challenges.

This cookbook is designed to make your culinary journey enjoyable and stress-free while supporting your kidney health. Embrace the delicious recipes and practical advice to maintain a healthy and fulfilling lifestyle.

TABLE OF CONTENTS

INTRODUCTION 2
   1.1 Understanding Stage 3 Kidney Disease 6
   1.2 Importance of Diet in Kidney Health 7
   1.3 Symptoms and Diagnosis 9

Chapter 1: Nutritional Guidelines for Stage 3 Kidney Disease 13
   2.1 Protein Management 13
   2.2 Sodium and Potassium Intake 16
   2.3 Phosphorus Control 19
   2.4 Fluid Restrictions 22

Chapter 2: Meal Planning and Preparation Tips 25
   3.1 Creating a Balanced Meal Plan 25
   3.2 Grocery Shopping Tips 29
   3.3 Cooking Techniques for Kidney Health 31

Chapter 3: Breakfast Recipes 34
   4.1 Low-Phosphorus Pancakes 34
   4.2 Kidney-Friendly Smoothies 36
   4.3 Vegetable Omelette 38
   4.4 Apple Cinnamon Oatmeal 40
   4.5 Blueberry Muffins 42
   4.6 Avocado Toast 44
   4.7 Banana Nut Bread 46
   4.8 Scrambled Tofu 48
   4.9 Greek Yogurt Parfait 50
   4.10 Cinnamon Quinoa 51
   4.11 Sweet Potato Hash 53
   4.12 Mango Chia Pudding 55
   4.13 Cottage Cheese and Peaches 57

    4.14 Spinach and Feta Wrap 59

Chapter 4: Lunch Recipes 61

    5.1 Quinoa and Vegetable Salad 61

    5.2 Grilled Chicken Wraps 63

    5.3 Lentil Soup 65

    5.4 Stuffed Bell Peppers 67

    5.5 Tuna Salad 69

    5.6 Chicken Caesar Salad 71

    5.7 Vegetable Stir-Fry 73

    5.8 Turkey and Avocado Sandwich 75

    5.9 Tomato Basil Soup 77

    5.10 Spinach and Mushroom Quiche 79

    5.11 Couscous Salad 81

    5.12 Chicken and Rice Bowl 83

    5.13 Veggie Burger 85

    5.14 Mediterranean Chickpea Salad 87

Chapter 5: Dinner Recipes 89

    6.1 Baked Salmon with Herbs 89

    6.2 Turkey and Vegetable Stir-Fry 91

    6.3 Spaghetti Squash with Marinara 93

    6.4 Beef and Broccoli 95

    6.5 Chicken Alfredo with Zoodles 97

    6.6 Grilled Shrimp Tacos 99

    6.7 Quinoa Stuffed Peppers 101

    6.8 Lemon Herb Chicken 103

    6.9 Vegetable Lasagna 105

    6.10 Herb-Crusted Tilapia 108

    6.11 Balsamic Glazed Pork Chops 110

    6.12 Stuffed Eggplant 112

    6.13 Ratatouille 114

    6.14 Moroccan Lentil Stew..116

Chapter 6: Snack and Appetizer Recipes..**118**
    7.1 Hummus with Fresh Vegetables..118
    7.2 Greek Yogurt with Berries..120
    7.3 Roasted Chickpeas...121
    7.4 Avocado Toast...124
    7.5 Apple Slices with Peanut Butter..126
    7.6 Cucumber Sandwiches...128
    7.7 Edamame...129
    7.8 Rice Cakes with Almond Butter..132
    7.9 Vegetable Spring Rolls..133
    7.10 Cheese and Crackers...137
    7.11 Popcorn with Nutritional Yeast...139
    7.12 Fruit Salad...141
    7.13 Kale Chips...142
    7.14 Deviled Eggs...145

Chapter 7: Dessert Recipes...**147**
    8.1 Berry Parfait..147
    8.2 Rice Pudding...149
    8.3 Low-Sugar Apple Crisp...151
    8.4 Coconut Macaroons...153
    8.5 Chia Seed Pudding..155
    8.6 Lemon Sorbet..156
    8.7 Banana Ice Cream...158
    8.8 Chocolate Avocado Mousse..160
    8.9 Peach Cobbler...162
    8.10 Pineapple Upside-Down Cake..164
    8.11 Oatmeal Cookies...167
    8.12 Strawberry Shortcake..169
    8.13 Almond Flour Brownies..172

    8.14 Carrot Cake.. 174

Chapter 8: Beverage Recipes... 177

    9.1 Herbal Teas... 177

    9.2 Infused Water..178

    9.3 Kidney-Friendly Smoothies... 181

    9.4 Low-Sugar Lemonade.. 183

    9.5 Green Juice..184

    9.6 Iced Tea... 185

    9.7 Coconut Water.. 188

    9.8 Almond Milk Shake.. 190

    9.9 Berry Blast Smoothie... 192

    9.10 Ginger Tea...194

    9.11 Cucumber Mint Water..196

    9.12 Apple Cinnamon Water... 198

    9.13 Chamomile Tea... 200

    9.14 Turmeric Latte.. 202

Chapter 9: Special Diets and Adjustments.. 204

    10.1 Vegetarian and Vegan Options...204

    10.2 Adjusting Recipes for Diabetic Patients....................................204

Chapter 10: Managing Dietary Challenges....................................... 206

    11.1 Overcoming Appetite Loss.. 206

    11.2 Managing Nausea and Vomiting.. 206

    11.3 Dealing with Dietary Restrictions.. 208

1.1 Understanding Stage 3 Kidney Disease

Stage 3 kidney disease is a crucial phase in the progression of chronic kidney disease (CKD), characterized by moderate damage to the kidneys. At this stage, the kidneys are functioning at approximately 30-59% of their normal capacity, as measured by the glomerular filtration rate (GFR). Understanding this stage is vital for managing your health and slowing the progression of the disease.

What Happens in Stage 3 Kidney Disease?
The kidneys' primary function is to filter waste and excess fluids from the blood, which are then excreted as urine. When the kidneys are damaged, they lose their ability to perform this function effectively. In Stage 3 CKD, waste products begin to build up in the blood, which can lead to a variety of health issues, including high blood pressure, anemia, and bone disease.

Importance of Early Detection and Management
Early detection of Stage 3 kidney disease is critical for preventing further progression to more severe stages. Regular check-ups with your healthcare provider, including blood tests and urine tests, can help monitor kidney function and detect any changes early on.

Managing Stage 3 kidney disease involves a combination of medical treatment, lifestyle changes, and dietary modifications. Your healthcare provider may recommend medications to control blood pressure, blood sugar, and cholesterol levels. Additionally, adopting a kidney-friendly diet is essential to reduce the workload on your kidneys and maintain overall health.

By understanding Stage 3 kidney disease and making informed lifestyle and dietary choices, you can take proactive steps to manage your condition and improve your quality of life.

1.2 Importance of Diet in Kidney Health

Diet is a cornerstone of managing kidney health, particularly for individuals with Stage 3 kidney disease. The right dietary choices can significantly impact the progression of the disease, help control symptoms, and improve overall well-being. Understanding the importance of diet in kidney health empowers you to make informed decisions that support your kidneys' function and enhance your quality of life.

Reducing Kidney Workload
One of the primary goals of a kidney-friendly diet is to reduce the workload on the kidneys. When kidneys are damaged, they struggle to filter waste and excess fluids from the blood. By carefully selecting the foods you eat, you can minimize the accumulation of waste products and reduce the strain on your kidneys. This is particularly important in Stage 3 kidney disease, where kidney function is already compromised.

Controlling Blood Pressure and Blood Sugar
High blood pressure and diabetes are leading causes of kidney disease. A diet low in sodium, refined sugars, and unhealthy fats can help control blood pressure and blood sugar levels, preventing further damage to the kidneys. By choosing whole, nutrient-dense foods and avoiding processed foods, you can better manage these conditions and support your kidney health.

Preventing Complications
A well-planned kidney-friendly diet helps prevent complications associated with kidney disease, such as bone disorders, anemia, and cardiovascular issues. By maintaining balanced nutrient levels, you can reduce the risk of these complications and improve your overall health.

Enhancing Quality of Life

Eating a balanced diet that supports kidney health can improve your energy levels, reduce symptoms, and enhance your overall quality of life. Enjoying a variety of delicious, kidney-friendly foods ensures that you get the nutrients you need while minimizing the risk of further kidney damage. This can help you stay active, engaged, and positive throughout your journey with kidney disease.

Diet plays a pivotal role in managing Stage 3 kidney disease. By making mindful food choices and working with healthcare professionals, you can take control of your kidney health, slow the progression of the disease, and lead a fulfilling, healthy life.

1.3 Symptoms and Diagnosis

Stage 3 kidney disease is often a critical juncture in the progression of chronic kidney disease (CKD), marked by moderate kidney damage and a significant reduction in kidney function. While many individuals may not experience obvious symptoms at this stage, it's important to recognize the signs that indicate worsening kidney health. Common symptoms include:

- **Fatigue and Weakness:** Reduced kidney function can lead to an accumulation of toxins and waste products in the blood, causing feelings of tiredness and weakness.
- **Swelling (Edema):** Fluid retention, particularly in the legs, ankles, feet, and hands, occurs due to the kidneys' impaired ability to balance fluid levels.
- Changes in Urination: You may notice changes in the frequency, color, and volume of urine. This can include more frequent urination, especially at night, or urine that appears foamy or bubbly.
- Shortness of Breath: Accumulation of excess fluid in the body can affect the lungs, leading to shortness of breath, particularly during physical activity or when lying down.
- Muscle Cramps: Imbalances in electrolytes, such as calcium and potassium, can cause muscle cramps and twitches.
- Insomnia: Difficulty sleeping can be a result of toxin buildup, restless legs, or muscle cramps.
- Dry and Itchy Skin: The buildup of waste products in the blood can cause skin dryness and itching.
- Nausea and Vomiting: Accumulation of toxins can lead to gastrointestinal symptoms such as nausea, vomiting, and loss of appetite.

It is important to note that symptoms can vary widely among individuals, and some people may not experience any noticeable symptoms at all. This is why regular monitoring and check-ups with a healthcare provider are crucial for early detection and management of the disease.

Diagnosis of Stage 3 Kidney Disease

Early diagnosis of Stage 3 kidney disease is vital for effective management and slowing the progression of the disease. Healthcare providers use a combination of methods to diagnose and monitor kidney function:

- ❖ **Medical History and Physical Examination:** Your doctor will begin by taking a thorough medical history, including any symptoms you may be experiencing, and performing a physical examination. This helps identify risk factors and signs of kidney disease.

- ❖ **Blood Tests:** Blood tests are essential for evaluating kidney function and identifying any imbalances in the body. Key blood tests include:

1. Serum Creatinine: Measures the level of creatinine in your blood. Elevated levels indicate reduced kidney function.

2. Estimated Glomerular Filtration Rate (eGFR): Calculated using serum creatinine, age, sex, and other factors, eGFR estimates how well your kidneys are filtering waste from the blood. A value of 30-59 mL/min/1.73 m^2 indicates Stage 3 kidney disease.

3. Blood Urea Nitrogen (BUN): Measures the amount of nitrogen in your blood that comes from the waste product urea. Elevated BUN levels can indicate kidney dysfunction.

4. Electrolytes and Minerals: Tests for levels of sodium, potassium, calcium, and phosphorus to identify imbalances that can occur with kidney disease.

- ❖ Urine Tests: Urine tests help assess kidney function and detect abnormalities. Important urine tests include:

1. Urinalysis: Analyzes the content of your urine for signs of kidney disease, such as protein or blood.

2. Urine Albumin-to-Creatinine Ratio (UACR): Measures the amount of albumin (a type of protein) in your urine. Elevated levels of albumin can indicate kidney damage.

- ❖ Imaging Tests: Imaging tests provide detailed pictures of your kidneys to identify structural abnormalities or blockages. Common imaging tests include:

1. Ultrasound: Uses sound waves to create images of your kidneys, helping to detect any abnormalities in size, shape, or structure.

2. CT Scan (Computed Tomography): Provides cross-sectional images of your kidneys to identify structural issues or blockages.

- ❖ Kidney Biopsy: In some cases, a kidney biopsy may be necessary to determine the extent of kidney damage. This includes taking a little example of kidney tissue for tiny assessment.

Regular Monitoring and Follow-up

Once diagnosed with Stage 3 kidney disease, regular monitoring and follow-up with your healthcare provider are crucial. This includes:

- Routine Blood and Urine Tests: To track kidney function and detect any changes early.
- Blood Pressure Monitoring: To ensure blood pressure is well-controlled, as hypertension can worsen kidney damage.
- Medications: Your doctor may prescribe medications to control blood pressure, blood sugar, and cholesterol levels to protect your kidneys.
- Dietary and Lifestyle Modifications: Following a kidney-friendly diet and adopting a healthy lifestyle to support kidney function.

Early diagnosis and proactive management of Stage 3 kidney disease can significantly slow its progression and improve your quality of life. By working closely with your healthcare team and adhering to recommended treatments and lifestyle changes, you can take control of your kidney health and reduce the risk of complications.

Chapter 1: Nutritional Guidelines for Stage 3 Kidney Disease

2.1 Protein Management

Protein is a vital nutrient for overall health, playing essential roles in building and repairing tissues, producing enzymes and hormones, and maintaining muscle mass. However, in Stage 3 kidney disease, managing protein intake becomes crucial to prevent additional stress on the kidneys and to manage waste products effectively.

The Role of Protein in Kidney Health

In Stage 3 kidney disease, the kidneys are functioning at a reduced capacity, which affects their ability to filter out waste products from protein metabolism. Excessive protein intake can lead to an accumulation of these waste products in the blood, increasing the workload on the kidneys and potentially accelerating the progression of the disease.

Determining Your Protein Needs

1. Assessing Protein Requirements:

- Individualized Goals: Protein needs vary depending on factors such as body weight, level of physical activity, and overall health. A renal dietitian can help determine the optimal amount of protein for your specific condition.
- General Recommendations: Typically, protein intake is moderated to about 0.6 to 0.8 grams per kilogram of body weight per day for individuals with Stage 3 kidney disease. However, this may vary based on individual needs and recommendations from your healthcare provider.

Practical Strategies for Managing Protein Intake

1. Portion Control:

- Balanced Portions: Consume appropriate portion sizes to manage protein intake effectively. For example, a serving of meat, poultry, or fish should be about 3 ounces, which is roughly the size of a deck of cards.
- Spread Out Intake: Distribute protein consumption evenly throughout the day to reduce the strain on your kidneys and aid in better utilization of protein.

2. Choose Kidney-Friendly Protein Sources:

- Lean Meats: Opt for lean cuts of beef, pork, or lamb, and remove visible fat and skin from poultry.
- Fish: Include fish such as salmon, trout, and tilapia, which provide high-quality protein and beneficial omega-3 fatty acids.
- Eggs: Eggs are a good source of high-quality protein and can be included in your diet in moderation.
- Plant-Based Proteins: Incorporate plant-based proteins like tofu, tempeh, and edamame, which offer essential amino acids with less strain on the kidneys compared to animal proteins.

3. Monitor and Adjust Protein Intake:

- Track Your Intake: Keep a food diary to monitor your daily protein consumption and make necessary adjustments based on your dietitian's recommendations.
- Regular Check-ups: Regularly review your protein intake with your healthcare provider or dietitian to ensure it aligns with your kidney health goals and adjust as needed.

Potential Risks of Excessive Protein

1. Increased Kidney Workload:

- Waste Product Accumulation: Excessive protein can lead to a buildup of urea and other waste products in the blood, which the kidneys must filter, potentially leading to further kidney damage.
- Fluid Imbalance: High protein intake can also affect fluid balance and increase the risk of dehydration.

2. Nutritional Imbalances:

- Potential Deficiencies: Excessive protein might lead to inadequate intake of other essential nutrients, such as carbohydrates and fats, which are also important for overall health.

Working with a Dietitian

Collaborating with a renal dietitian is essential for effective protein management. A dietitian can help:

- Create a Personalized Plan: Develop a meal plan that meets your protein needs while considering other dietary restrictions and preferences.
- Provide Education: Offer guidance on selecting appropriate protein sources, portion sizes, and meal planning.
- Monitor Progress: Regularly review and adjust your protein intake based on your kidney function, symptoms, and overall health.

By carefully managing your protein intake, you can help reduce the strain on your kidneys, prevent complications, and maintain a balanced diet that supports your health and well-being.

2.2 Sodium and Potassium Intake

Managing sodium and potassium intake is crucial for individuals with Stage 3 kidney disease. Both minerals play essential roles in maintaining fluid balance, blood pressure, and overall health. However, impaired kidney function can make it challenging to regulate these minerals, necessitating careful dietary management.

Sodium Intake

Importance: Sodium is a key mineral that helps regulate fluid balance, blood pressure, and nerve function. However, excessive sodium intake can lead to fluid retention, increased blood pressure, and further strain on the kidneys. This is especially problematic in Stage 3 kidney disease, where fluid balance and blood pressure control are already compromised.

Recommended Intake:

- **Limit Sodium:** The general recommendation for sodium intake is to consume less than 2,300 milligrams per day. For individuals with kidney disease, a lower target may be advised by your healthcare provider, often around 1,500 to 2,000 milligrams per day.

Practical Tips:

- **Avoid Processed Foods:** Processed and packaged foods often contain high amounts of sodium. Limit or avoid items such as canned soups, frozen dinners, and salty snacks.
- **Read Labels:** Continuously check sustenance marks for sodium content. Look for products labeled "low sodium" or "no added salt."
- **Flavor with Herbs and Spices:** Enhance the flavor of your meals using herbs, spices, garlic, and vinegar instead of salt.

- **Cook Fresh Foods:** Prepare meals from fresh ingredients whenever possible. Cooking at home allows you to control the amount of sodium added to your dishes.

Potassium Intake

Importance: Potassium is essential for maintaining normal muscle function, nerve function, and heart rhythm. However, in Stage 3 kidney disease, the kidneys may struggle to maintain proper potassium levels, leading to potential imbalances. Elevated potassium levels (hyperkalemia) can be dangerous and lead to serious heart problems.

Recommended Intake:

- **Monitor Potassium:** The appropriate amount of potassium varies depending on individual needs and kidney function. A common target is to limit potassium intake to about 2,000 to 3,000 milligrams per day, but this should be personalized based on your blood test results and advice from your healthcare provider.

Practical Tips:

- **Limit High-Potassium Foods:** Reduce intake of foods high in potassium, such as bananas, oranges, potatoes, tomatoes, and spinach.
- **Choose Lower-Potassium Alternatives:** Opt for fruits and vegetables lower in potassium, such as apples, berries, carrots, and green beans.
- **Leach Vegetables:** Leaching is a method to reduce potassium levels in vegetables. Boil chopped vegetables and discard the water, then cook with fresh water to further reduce potassium content.
- **Monitor Portion Sizes:** Pay attention to portion sizes of potassium-rich foods, even if you choose to include them occasionally.

Balancing Sodium and Potassium

1. Fluid Balance: Both sodium and potassium affect fluid balance in the body. Managing your intake of these minerals helps control swelling, fluid retention, and blood pressure.

2. Blood Pressure Management: Sodium reduction helps lower blood pressure, while potassium can assist in maintaining healthy blood pressure levels. Balancing both minerals is essential for overall cardiovascular health.

3. Regular Monitoring: Regular blood tests are necessary to monitor sodium and potassium levels. Your healthcare provider will use these results to adjust your dietary recommendations and ensure that both minerals are within a safe range.

Working with a Healthcare Provider

1. Personalized Guidance: Collaborate with a renal dietitian or healthcare provider to tailor sodium and potassium recommendations to your specific needs. They can help you understand your dietary restrictions and provide practical advice on managing these minerals.

2. Dietary Adjustments: Based on your test results and health status, your dietitian can help you make necessary adjustments to your diet, including choosing appropriate foods and managing portion sizes.

3. Monitor Symptoms: Be aware of symptoms related to sodium and potassium imbalances, such as swelling, high blood pressure, muscle cramps, or irregular heart rhythms. Report any surprising side effects to your medical care supplier immediately

By carefully managing your sodium and potassium intake, you can support kidney function, prevent complications, and maintain better overall health.

2.3 Phosphorus Control

Phosphorus is an essential mineral that plays a crucial role in maintaining healthy bones and teeth, as well as in energy production and cell function. However, in Stage 3 kidney disease, managing phosphorus levels is vital because impaired kidney function can lead to an accumulation of phosphorus in the blood. Elevated phosphorus levels can contribute to bone and cardiovascular problems, making phosphorus control an important aspect of dietary management.

Importance of Phosphorus Control

1. Bone Health: Elevated phosphorus levels can lead to imbalances in calcium and phosphorus, which can result in weakened bones and an increased risk of fractures. This condition, known as renal osteodystrophy, is common in individuals with chronic kidney disease (CKD).

2. Cardiovascular Health: High phosphorus levels can contribute to the calcification of blood vessels and heart valves, increasing the risk of cardiovascular disease.

3. Secondary Hyperparathyroidism: Excess phosphorus can lead to increased parathyroid hormone (PTH) production, a condition known as secondary hyperparathyroidism. Elevated PTH can further exacerbate bone and mineral disorders.

Recommended Phosphorus Intake

1. General Guidelines: For individuals with Stage 3 kidney disease, it is typically recommended to limit phosphorus intake to about 800 to 1,000 milligrams per day. However, specific recommendations may vary based on individual needs and test results.

2. Phosphorus Monitoring: Regular blood tests are essential to monitor phosphorus levels and adjust dietary recommendations accordingly. Your healthcare provider will use these results to tailor your phosphorus management plan.

Practical Strategies for Phosphorus Control

1. Limit High-Phosphorus Foods:

- **Dairy Products:** Milk, cheese, yogurt, and other dairy products are high in phosphorus. Choose lower-phosphorus alternatives or limit portion sizes.
- **Nuts and Seeds:** Nuts, seeds, and nut butters contain high levels of phosphorus. Consume them in moderation or choose lower-phosphorus alternatives.
- **Whole Grains:** Whole grains like brown rice, oatmeal, and whole wheat bread have higher phosphorus content compared to refined grains. Opt for refined grains and limit whole grain intake.

2. Avoid Phosphorus Additives:

- **Processed Foods:** Many processed and packaged foods contain added phosphorus in the form of phosphate additives, which are absorbed more easily by the body. Avoid or limit foods with ingredients like phosphoric acid or sodium phosphate.
- **Read Labels:** Check food labels for phosphorus additives and choose products without these additives whenever possible.

3. Choose Phosphorus-Binding Medications:

- **Phosphate Binders:** Your healthcare provider may prescribe phosphate binders to help reduce phosphorus absorption from food. These medications should be taken as directed with meals to be effective.

4. Opt for Phosphorus-Lowering Foods:

- **Low-Phosphorus Alternatives:** Select foods that are lower in phosphorus, such as refined grains (white rice, white bread), certain fruits (apples, berries), and vegetables (green beans, cucumbers).
- **Cooking Methods:** Use cooking methods that can help reduce phosphorus content, such as boiling vegetables and discarding the water.

Working with a Dietitian

1. Personalized Dietary Plan: Collaborate with a renal dietitian to create a personalized meal plan that manages phosphorus intake while meeting your nutritional needs. The dietitian can provide guidance on choosing low-phosphorus foods and avoiding high-phosphorus options.

2. Education and Support: A dietitian can offer education on reading food labels, understanding ingredient lists, and making informed food choices to control phosphorus levels effectively.

3. Monitoring and Adjustments: Regular follow-ups with your dietitian can help monitor phosphorus levels and make necessary adjustments to your diet and treatment plan based on your health status.

Controlling phosphorus intake is crucial for managing Stage 3 kidney disease and preventing complications related to bone and cardiovascular health. By limiting high-phosphorus foods, avoiding phosphorus additives, and working closely with your healthcare provider and dietitian, you can effectively manage phosphorus levels and support your overall well-being.

2.4 Fluid Restrictions

Fluid management is a critical aspect of managing Stage 3 kidney disease. The kidneys play a vital role in regulating fluid balance in the body, but when kidney function is compromised, it becomes challenging to maintain this balance. Proper fluid management helps prevent complications such as fluid overload, swelling, high blood pressure, and shortness of breath.

Importance of Fluid Restrictions

1. Preventing Fluid Overload: Impaired kidney function can lead to fluid retention, causing swelling (edema) in the legs, ankles, feet, and hands. Excess fluid in the body can also accumulate in the lungs, leading to shortness of breath and discomfort.

2. Controlling Blood Pressure: Excessive fluid intake can increase blood volume, leading to higher blood pressure. Managing fluid intake helps control blood pressure, reducing the risk of cardiovascular complications.

3. Reducing Symptoms: Proper fluid management can alleviate symptoms such as swelling, weight gain, and difficulty breathing, improving overall comfort and quality of life.

Determining Fluid Needs

1. Individualized Recommendations: Fluid needs vary depending on individual health conditions, kidney function, and symptoms. Your healthcare provider will assess your specific needs and provide personalized fluid intake recommendations.

2. Typical Guidelines: While liquid necessities are individualized, a typical proposal for people with Stage 3 kidney sickness is to restrict liquid admission to around 1.5 to 2 liters each day, including all drinks and food varieties with high water content.

Practical Strategies for Fluid Restrictions

1. Monitor Fluid Intake:

- **Track Consumption:** Keep a daily record of all fluids consumed, including water, beverages, soups, and foods with high water content.
- **Use Measuring Tools:** Use measuring cups and bottles to help monitor and control portion sizes.

2. Manage Fluid Intake:

- **Distribute Throughout the Day:** Spread fluid consumption evenly throughout the day to avoid consuming large amounts at once, which can increase the risk of fluid overload.
- **Adjust Based on Activity:** Modify fluid intake based on physical activity levels, weather conditions, and individual needs. For example, you may need to adjust fluid intake on hot days or after exercise.

3. Choose Hydrating Foods Wisely:

- **Low-Water Content Foods:** Opt for foods with lower water content, such as dry snacks and foods prepared without added fluids.
- **Flavor Alternatives:** Use flavoring options like herbs, spices, or lemon juice to enhance the taste of your meals without adding extra fluid.

4. Limit High-Fluids Foods:

- **Soups and Stews:** Reduce consumption of soups, stews, and broths, as they contribute to total fluid intake.
- **Ice Cream and Popsicles:** Limit frozen treats that contain high amounts of water.

Dealing with Thirst

1. Hydration Tips:

- **Ice Chips:** Suck on ice chips or a small piece of fruit to help manage thirst without consuming large amounts of fluid.
- **Chewing Gum:** Chewing sugar-free gum can help reduce the sensation of thirst.

2. Address Underlying Causes:

- **Medication Side Effects:** If medications cause increased thirst or fluid retention, discuss alternatives or adjustments with your healthcare provider.
- **Dietary Adjustments:** Work with a dietitian to address any dietary factors contributing to increased thirst.

Working with Your Healthcare Provider

1. Personalized Plan: Collaborate with your healthcare provider to develop a fluid restriction plan tailored to your specific needs and health condition. Regular monitoring and adjustments are essential to ensure that fluid restrictions are effective and safe.

2. Monitor Symptoms: Keep track of symptoms related to fluid imbalance, such as swelling, shortness of breath, and weight gain. Report any progressions or worries to your medical services supplier instantly.

3. Regular Follow-ups: Schedule regular check-ups with your healthcare provider to assess fluid balance, kidney function, and overall health. Adjustments to fluid restrictions may be necessary based on these evaluations.

Effective fluid management is essential for individuals with Stage 3 kidney disease to prevent complications related to fluid overload, blood pressure, and overall comfort. By monitoring fluid intake, choosing hydrating foods wisely, managing thirst, and working closely with your healthcare provider, you can maintain optimal fluid balance and support your kidney health.

Chapter 2: Meal Planning and Preparation Tips

3.1 Creating a Balanced Meal Plan

Creating a balanced meal plan is essential for managing Stage 3 kidney disease and ensuring you get the necessary nutrients while adhering to dietary restrictions. A well-planned diet helps control symptoms, prevent complications, and support overall health. Here's how to develop a balanced meal plan tailored to your needs:

Understanding Your Nutritional Needs

1. Assessing Individual Requirements:

- **Protein:** Determine your protein needs based on your weight, level of physical activity, and kidney function. Typically, this involves moderate protein intake to reduce the workload on your kidneys.
- **Sodium, Potassium, and Phosphorus:** Follow guidelines for limiting sodium, potassium, and phosphorus based on your blood test results and healthcare provider's recommendations.
- **Fluid:** Manage fluid intake to prevent overload and associated complications.

2. Nutrient Distribution:

- **Macronutrients:** Balance your intake of carbohydrates, proteins, and fats. Carbohydrates provide energy, proteins support tissue repair, and fats are essential for overall health.
- **Micronutrients:** Ensure adequate intake of vitamins and minerals while adhering to restrictions on sodium, potassium, and phosphorus.

Designing Your Meal Plan

1. Plan Balanced Meals:

- **Breakfast:** Include a source of high-quality protein (e.g., eggs, lean meats) and pair it with low-potassium fruits (e.g., berries) and whole grains (e.g., white bread or rice).
- **Lunch:** Create a balanced meal with lean protein (e.g., grilled chicken), low-potassium vegetables (e.g., green beans, cucumbers), and a moderate portion of refined grains.
- **Dinner:** Opt for a protein source (e.g., fish), a side of low-potassium vegetables, and a serving of refined grains. Use spices and flavors for flavor rather than salt.

2. Incorporate Snacks:

- **Healthy Choices:** Choose low-sodium, low-potassium snacks such as apple slices, rice cakes, or unsalted crackers.
- **Portion Control:** Keep snack portions moderate to manage overall nutrient intake and fluid balance.

3. Use Cooking Methods Wisely:

- **Healthier Cooking Techniques:** Use methods like baking, grilling, or steaming instead of frying to reduce added fats and sodium.
- **Flavor Enhancements:** Enhance flavors with herbs, spices, garlic, and lemon juice instead of salt.

4. Create a Weekly Plan:

- **Variety:** Include a variety of foods to ensure a balanced intake of nutrients and prevent dietary monotony.
- **Meal Prep:** Prepare meals in advance to simplify meal planning and ensure adherence to dietary guidelines.

Managing Portion Sizes

1. Control Portions:

- **Protein:** Keep protein portions moderate, typically around 3 ounces per meal.
- **Carbohydrates and Fats:** Balance carbohydrate and fat intake to meet energy needs without overloading the kidneys.

2. Use Visual Cues:

- **Portion Guides:** Use visual aids or measuring tools to help manage portion sizes, such as comparing protein portions to the size of a deck of cards.

Adapting to Dietary Restrictions

1. Sodium Management:

- **Low-Sodium Alternatives:** Choose fresh or frozen vegetables, and avoid processed foods high in sodium.
- **Flavor without Salt:** Use salt-free seasoning blends and herbs to add flavor.

2. Potassium Management:

- **Low-Potassium Choices:** Opt for fruits and vegetables lower in potassium and monitor portion sizes.

3. Phosphorus Management:

- **Limit High-Phosphorus Foods:** Reduce intake of dairy products, nuts, and whole grains. Choose refined grains and foods without phosphorus additives.

4. Fluid Management:

- **Monitor Intake:** Track all sources of fluid, including beverages and high-water-content foods. Adjust portions based on individual needs.

Working with a Dietitian

1. Personalized Guidance:

- **Custom Meal Plans:** Work with a renal dietitian to create a meal plan tailored to your specific nutritional needs and dietary restrictions.
- **Education and Support:** A dietitian can provide education on food choices, portion sizes, and meal planning techniques.

2. Regular Monitoring:

- **Adjustments:** Regularly review and adjust your meal plan based on changes in your health, blood test results, and dietary needs.

3. Goal Setting:

- **Achieving Balance:** Set realistic goals for managing your diet and work with your dietitian to achieve and maintain a balanced meal plan.

Creating a balanced meal plan for Stage 3 kidney disease involves careful consideration of your nutritional needs and dietary restrictions. By planning balanced meals, managing portion sizes, using appropriate cooking methods, and working with a dietitian, you can support your kidney health and overall well-being while enjoying a varied and satisfying diet.

3.2 Grocery Shopping Tips

Fruits:

- Apples
- Berries (e.g., strawberries, blueberries)
- Peaches
- Grapes
- Pineapple

Vegetables:

- Carrots
- Green beans
- Cucumbers
- Bell peppers
- Cauliflower

Proteins:

- Chicken breast
- Turkey breast
- Fish (e.g., salmon, cod)
- Tofu
- Tempeh

Grains:

- White rice
- White bread
- Plain pasta
- Refined cereals (e.g., cornflakes)

Dairy Alternatives:

- Unsweetened almond milk
- Rice milk
- Low-phosphorus cheese (if allowed)

Low-Sodium Snacks:

- Unsalted rice cakes
- Fresh fruit
- Low-sodium crackers

Cooking Ingredients:

- Olive oil
- Herbs and spices (e.g., basil, thyme, rosemary)
- Garlic
- Vinegar (e.g., apple cider vinegar)

Beverages:

- Plain water
- Herbal teas (non-caffeinated)
- Sparkling water (unsweetened)

Condiments:

- Low-sodium soy sauce
- Lemon juice
- Salt-free seasoning blends

Frozen Foods:

- Frozen berries
- Frozen vegetables (e.g., green beans, peas)
- Frozen fish fillets

3.3 Cooking Techniques for Kidney Health

Using appropriate cooking techniques can help manage Stage 3 kidney disease by reducing sodium, potassium, phosphorus, and other potentially harmful components in your diet. Here are some kidney-friendly cooking methods and tips to help you prepare nutritious and delicious meals while adhering to dietary restrictions:

1. Steaming

- **Benefits:** Steaming helps retain the nutrients in vegetables and reduces the need for added fats or sodium.
- **How to Do It:** Use a steamer basket or a dedicated steamer appliance. Steam vegetables like carrots, green beans, and broccoli until tender.

2. Baking

- **Benefits:** Baking is a healthy method that requires little or no added fat. It can enhance flavors without extra sodium.
- **How to Do It:** Bake lean proteins (e.g., chicken breast, fish) and vegetables. Season with spices and flavors rather than salt.

3. Grilling

- **Benefits:** Grilling adds a smoky flavor to foods without using extra fat or sodium. It's ideal for lean meats and vegetables.
- **How to Do It:** Use a grill or grill pan. Marinate proteins with low-sodium options or use a salt-free seasoning blend.

4. Boiling and Blanching

- **Benefits:** Boiling and blanching can help reduce potassium content in vegetables.

- **How to Do It:** Boil chopped vegetables, then discard the water and cook with fresh water. Blanching involves briefly boiling vegetables, then plunging them into ice water to stop cooking.

5. Sautéing

- **Benefits:** Sautéing uses a small amount of oil and can enhance the flavor of foods without adding sodium.
- **How to Do It:** Use a non-stick pan with a small amount of olive oil. Sauté vegetables and proteins with herbs and spices.

6. Slow Cooking

- **Benefits:** Slow cooking allows flavors to develop without the need for excess salt. It's convenient for preparing large batches of meals.
- **How to Do It:** Use a slow cooker to prepare soups, stews, and casseroles. Opt for low-sodium broths and use fresh herbs for flavor.

7. Poaching

- **Benefits:** Poaching is a gentle cooking method that can help retain the moisture and nutrients in proteins like fish and poultry.
- **How to Do It:** Simmer proteins in a small amount of water or broth at a low temperature until cooked through.

8. Roasting

- **Benefits:** Roasting can bring out the natural sweetness of vegetables and add a crispy texture without excessive oil or sodium.
- **How to Do It:** Roast vegetables and lean meats in the oven. Use minimal olive oil and season with herbs and spices.

9. Microwaving

- **Benefits:** Microwaving is a quick and efficient method that helps retain nutrients and requires little or no added fat.
- **How to Do It:** Use microwave-safe dishes to cook vegetables, rice, and lean proteins. Avoid using high-sodium pre-packaged microwave meals.

10. Pressure Cooking

- **Benefits:** Pressure cooking can reduce cooking time and help retain nutrients while minimizing the need for added fats or sodium.
- **How to Do It:** Use a pressure cooker or Instant Pot to prepare soups, stews, and grains quickly and efficiently.

Additional Tips for Kidney-Friendly Cooking:

- **Use Low-Sodium Ingredients:** Choose low-sodium or no-salt-added versions of sauces, broths, and canned goods.
- **Flavor with Herbs and Spices:** Enhance the taste of your dishes with herbs, spices, garlic, and vinegar instead of salt.
- **Rinse Canned Foods:** If using canned vegetables or beans, rinse them thoroughly to remove excess sodium.
- **Portion Control:** Be mindful of portion sizes to manage protein, sodium, and phosphorus intake effectively.

Employing kidney-friendly cooking techniques can significantly impact your health and dietary management in Stage 3 kidney disease. By using methods such as steaming, baking, grilling, and sautéing, you can prepare delicious and nutritious meals that align with your dietary restrictions. Incorporating these techniques helps reduce the need for added fats and sodium while preserving the natural flavors and nutrients of your foods.

Chapter 3: Breakfast Recipes

4.1 Low-Phosphorus Pancakes

Ingredients

- 1 cup all-purpose flour
- 1 tablespoon granulated sugar
- 2 teaspoons baking powder
- 1/8 teaspoon salt
- 2 large egg whites
- 1 cup 1% low-fat milk (or a phosphorus-free alternative like almond milk)
- 2 tablespoons canola oil

Directions

1. **Mix Dry Ingredients**: In a medium bowl, combine the flour, sugar, baking powder, and salt.
2. **Prepare Wet Ingredients**: In a separate large bowl, whisk together the egg whites, milk, and canola oil.
3. **Combine Mixtures**: Pour the wet ingredients into the dry ingredients all at once. Stir until just moistened; the batter should remain lumpy.
4. **Heat the Griddle**: Preheat a lightly greased griddle or skillet over medium heat.
5. **Cook Pancakes**: Pour about 1/4 cup of batter onto the hot griddle for each pancake. Cook for about 2 minutes on each side or until golden brown. Flip the pancakes when bubbles form on the surface and the edges appear dry.
6. **Serve**: Enjoy the pancakes warm, optionally topped with fruits, syrup, or a non-dairy spread.

Cooking and Prep Time

- **Prep Time**: 15 minutes
- **Cook Time**: 20 minutes

- **Total Time**: 35 minutes

Servings

This recipe makes about 4 servings (2 pancakes per serving).

Nutritional Information (per serving)

- **Calories**: 178
- **Protein**: 6 g
- **Carbohydrates**: 25 g
- **Fat**: 6 g
- **Saturated Fat**: 1 g
- **Sodium**: 297 mg
- **Potassium**: 126 mg
- **Phosphorus**: 116 mg
- **Calcium**: 174 mg
- **Fiber**: 0.7 g

4.2 Kidney-Friendly Smoothies

Ingredients

- **1/2 cup strawberries** (fresh or frozen)
- **1/4 cup raspberries** (fresh or frozen)
- **1/4 cup blackberries** (fresh or frozen)
- **1/2 cup almond milk** (unsweetened)
- **1 handful baby spinach** (optional for added nutrients)
- **1 tablespoon honey or maple syrup** (optional for sweetness)

Directions

1. **Prepare Ingredients**: Wash the berries and spinach thoroughly. If using fresh berries, remove any stems.
2. **Blend**: In a blender, combine the strawberries, raspberries, blackberries, almond milk, and spinach. If desired, add honey or maple syrup for sweetness.
3. **Blend Until Smooth**: Blend on high speed until the mixture is smooth and creamy. If the smoothie is too thick, add a little more almond milk until the desired consistency is reached.
4. **Serve**: Pour the smoothie into a glass and enjoy immediately. Optionally, garnish with fresh berries on top.

Cooking and Prep Time

- **Prep Time**: 10 minutes
- **Total Time**: 10 minutes

Servings

This recipe yields approximately 1 serving.

Nutritional Information (per serving)

- **Calories**: 191
- **Protein**: 4 g
- **Carbohydrates**: 40.9 g

- **Fat**: 3.5 g
- **Sodium**: 143 mg
- **Potassium**: 679 mg
- **Phosphorus**: ~76.6 mg
- **Calcium**: 387 mg
- **Fiber**: 12.7 g

4.3 Vegetable Omelette

Ingredients

- 2 large eggs
- 3 shallots, sliced thinly
- 1 small green chili, chopped finely
- 1 small tomato, chopped finely
- 1 medium carrot, grated
- 3 tablespoons fresh coriander leaves (cilantro), chopped
- 1/2 teaspoon chili powder
- 1/2 teaspoon pepper powder
- 1/2 teaspoon turmeric powder
- Salt to taste
- 1 tablespoon oil (vegetable or olive oil)

Directions

1. **Prepare the Egg Mixture**: In a bowl, combine the eggs, shallots, green chili, tomato, grated carrot, coriander leaves, chili powder, pepper powder, turmeric powder, and salt. Beat the mixture until well combined.
2. **Heat the Pan**: Heat the oil in a non-stick pan over medium heat.
3. **Cook the Omelette**: Pour the egg mixture into the pan. Cook for about 2-3 minutes, or until the edges start to set.
4. **Flip the Omelette**: Place a plate over the pan and carefully flip the omelette onto the plate. Slide it back into the pan to cook the other side for an additional 2 minutes, or until fully cooked.
5. **Serve**: Remove the omelette from the pan and serve hot. You can garnish it with additional coriander leaves if desired.

Cooking and Prep Time

- **Prep Time**: 10 minutes

- **Cook Time**: 5-7 minutes
- **Total Time**: 15-17 minutes

Servings

This recipe makes approximately 1 serving.

Nutritional Information (per serving)

- **Calories**: 130 kcal
- **Protein**: 6 g
- **Carbohydrates**: 1 g
- **Fat**: 11 g
- **Saturated Fat**: 2 g
- **Cholesterol**: 164 mg
- **Sodium**: 71 mg
- **Potassium**: 93 mg
- **Fiber**: 0.4 g
- **Sugar**: 0.3 g
- **Vitamin A**: 594 IU
- **Calcium**: 28 mg
- **Iron**: 1 mg

4.4 Apple Cinnamon Oatmeal

Ingredients

- 1 medium apple, peeled and diced
- 1 tablespoon butter (or margarine)
- 1 cup water
- 1/2 cup milk (or a dairy-free alternative)
- 1/4 teaspoon salt
- 3/4 cup old-fashioned rolled oats
- 2 teaspoons ground cinnamon
- 2 tablespoons brown sugar (adjust to taste)
- 1 tablespoon white sugar (optional)
- 1/2 teaspoon nutmeg (optional)

Directions

1. **Sauté the Apple**: In a medium saucepan, melt the butter over medium heat. Add the diced apple and cook for about 3 minutes until slightly softened.
2. **Add Liquids**: Pour in the water, milk, and salt. Bring the mixture to a boil.
3. **Add Oats and Spices**: Once boiling, stir in the oats, cinnamon, nutmeg, and sugars. Mix well to combine.
4. **Cook the Oatmeal**: Reduce the heat to low and simmer for about 5-7 minutes, stirring occasionally, until the oatmeal reaches your desired consistency.
5. **Serve**: Spoon the oatmeal into bowls and top with additional cinnamon or a sprinkle of brown sugar if desired.

Cooking and Prep Time

- **Prep Time**: 5 minutes
- **Cook Time**: 10 minutes
- **Total Time**: 15 minutes

Servings

This recipe makes approximately 2 servings.

Nutritional Information (per serving)

- **Calories**: 180 kcal
- **Protein**: 5 g
- **Carbohydrates**: 37 g
- **Fat**: 2 g
- **Saturated Fat**: 1 g
- **Sodium**: 244 mg
- **Potassium**: 235 mg
- **Fiber**: 6 g
- **Sugar**: 12 g
- **Vitamin A**: 60 IU
- **Calcium**: 31 mg
- **Iron**: 2 mg

4.5 Blueberry Muffins

Ingredients

- 1 1/2 cups all-purpose flour
- 3/4 cup granulated sugar, plus 1 tablespoon for muffin tops
- 2 teaspoons baking powder
- 1/4 teaspoon salt
- 1/3 cup neutral-flavored oil (such as safflower, avocado, or vegetable oil)
- 1 large egg
- 1/3 cup milk or non-dairy milk
- 1 1/2 teaspoons vanilla extract
- 6-8 ounces fresh or frozen blueberries (generous 1 cup)

Directions

1. **Preheat the oven** to 400°F (204°C). Line a 12-count muffin pan with paper liners or grease the cups.
2. **In a large bowl, whisk together** the flour, 3/4 cup sugar, baking powder, and salt.
3. **In a separate bowl, whisk together** the oil, egg, milk, and vanilla.
4. **Pour the wet ingredients** into the dry ingredients and stir just until combined (do not overmix). Gently fold in the blueberries.
5. **Spoon the batter** into the prepared muffin cups, filling them all the way to the top.
6. **Sprinkle the remaining 1 tablespoon of sugar** evenly over the muffin tops.
7. **Bake for 5 minutes at 400°F**, then reduce the oven temperature to 350°F (177°C) and continue baking for 13-15 minutes, until a toothpick inserted in the center comes out clean.
8. **Allow the muffins to cool in the pan** for 5 minutes before transferring to a wire rack to cool completely.

Cooking and Prep Time

- **Prep Time**: 10 minutes
- **Cook Time**: 18-20 minutes
- **Total Time**: 28-30 minutes

Servings

This recipe makes 10-12 standard-sized muffins.

Nutritional Information (per muffin)

- Calories: 200
- Total Fat: 8 g
- Saturated Fat: 1 g
- Cholesterol: 25 mg
- Sodium: 210 mg
- Total Carbohydrates: 30 g
- Dietary Fiber: 1 g
- Total Sugars: 16 g
- Protein: 3 g

4.6 Avocado Toast

Ingredients

- 1 ripe avocado
- 1-2 slices of bread (sourdough, whole grain, or your choice)
- 1/2 lemon (for juice)
- Salt and pepper (to taste)
- Red pepper flakes (optional, for heat)
- Extra-virgin olive oil (for drizzling)
- Optional toppings: sliced tomatoes, radishes, poached egg, feta cheese, or fresh herbs

Directions

1. **Toast the Bread**: Start by toasting your slices of bread until golden brown and crispy.
2. **Prepare the Avocado**: While the bread is toasting, cut the avocado in half, remove the pit, and scoop the flesh into a bowl. Add the juice of half a lemon, salt, and pepper. Mash the avocado with a fork to your desired consistency (smooth or chunky).
3. **Assemble the Toast**: Once the bread is toasted, spread the mashed avocado generously on top of each slice.
4. **Add Toppings**: Drizzle with extra-virgin olive oil and sprinkle with red pepper flakes if desired. You can also add any optional toppings you like.
5. **Serve**: Enjoy immediately while the toast is warm.

Cooking and Prep Time

- **Prep Time**: 5 minutes
- **Cook Time**: 3-5 minutes (for toasting)
- **Total Time**: 8-10 minutes

Servings

This recipe serves 1-2, depending on the number of slices used.

Nutritional Information (per slice with avocado)

- **Calories**: Approximately 200-250 kcal (depending on bread type and toppings)
- **Protein**: 4 g
- **Carbohydrates**: 28 g
- **Fat**: 10-15 g (mostly healthy fats from avocado)
- **Saturated Fat**: 1-2 g
- **Sodium**: 150 mg (varies with added salt)
- **Fiber**: 6 g

4.7 Banana Nut Bread

Ingredients

- 1 ½ cups all-purpose flour
- 1 teaspoon baking soda
- ½ teaspoon ground cinnamon (optional)
- ¼ teaspoon salt
- ½ cup butter, softened
- ¾ cup granulated sugar
- 2 large eggs, room temperature
- 2 cups mashed bananas (about 4 medium ripe bananas)
- 1 teaspoon vanilla extract
- ¾ cup chopped walnuts (or pecans)

Directions

1. **Preheat the Oven**: Preheat your oven to 350°F (175°C). Grease a 9x5 inch loaf pan or line it with parchment paper.
2. **Mix Dry Ingredients**: In a medium bowl, whisk together the flour, baking soda, cinnamon (if using), and salt. Set aside.
3. **Cream Butter and Sugar**: In a large mixing bowl, beat the softened butter and sugar together until smooth and creamy.
4. **Add Eggs and Bananas**: Add the eggs one at a time, mixing well after each addition. Then, beat in the mashed bananas and vanilla extract until fully combined.
5. **Combine Mixtures**: Gradually add the dry ingredients to the wet mixture, stirring gently until just combined. Be careful not to overmix. Fold in the chopped walnuts.
6. **Bake**: Pour the batter into the prepared loaf pan. Bake for 55-60 minutes, or until a toothpick inserted into the center comes out clean.

7. **Cool**: Allow the bread to cool in the pan for about 10 minutes before transferring it to a wire rack to cool completely.

Cooking and Prep Time

- **Prep Time**: 10 minutes
- **Cook Time**: 55-60 minutes
- **Total Time**: 1 hour 5-10 minutes

Servings

This recipe yields approximately 10 servings.

Nutritional Information (per slice)

- **Calories**: 319 kcal
- **Protein**: 4 g
- **Carbohydrates**: 45 g
- **Fat**: 14 g
- **Saturated Fat**: 8 g
- **Cholesterol**: 43 mg
- **Sodium**: 210 mg
- **Potassium**: 200 mg
- **Fiber**: 1.5 g
- **Sugar**: 15 g

4.8 Scrambled Tofu

Ingredients

- 1 (14-16 ounce) block firm or extra-firm tofu
- 1 tablespoon olive oil (or any cooking oil)
- 1/2 medium onion, diced
- 2-3 cloves garlic, minced
- 1/4 teaspoon ground turmeric (for color)
- 1 tablespoon nutritional yeast (optional, for a cheesy flavor)
- Salt and pepper (to taste)
- 1/4 teaspoon garlic powder (optional)
- 1/4 teaspoon paprika (optional)
- Fresh vegetables (such as spinach, bell peppers, or tomatoes, optional)
- Fresh herbs (like parsley or cilantro, for garnish, optional)

Directions

1. **Prepare the Tofu**: Drain the tofu and press it to remove excess moisture. Wrap the tofu in a clean kitchen towel or paper towels, place it on a plate, and weigh it down with a heavy object for about 10-15 minutes.
2. **Sauté the Aromatics**: In a large skillet, heat the olive oil over medium heat. Add the diced onion and sauté for about 5 minutes until translucent. Add the minced garlic and cook for an additional minute until fragrant.
3. **Crumble the Tofu**: Once the tofu is pressed, crumble it into the skillet using your hands or a fork, breaking it into small pieces resembling scrambled eggs.
4. **Season the Tofu**: Sprinkle the turmeric, nutritional yeast, salt, pepper, garlic powder, and paprika over the crumbled tofu. Stir well to combine and cook for about 5-7 minutes, allowing the tofu to absorb the flavors.
5. **Add Vegetables**: If using vegetables, add them to the skillet and cook for an additional 2-3 minutes until they are tender.

6. **Serve**: Taste and adjust the seasoning if necessary. Serve the scrambled tofu warm, garnished with fresh herbs if desired. It pairs well with toast, in a wrap, or on its own.

Cooking and Prep Time

- **Prep Time**: 15 minutes
- **Cook Time**: 10-15 minutes
- **Total Time**: 25-30 minutes

Servings

This recipe serves approximately 2-3 people.

Nutritional Information (per serving)

- **Calories**: 180 kcal
- **Protein**: 16 g
- **Carbohydrates**: 6 g
- **Fat**: 10 g
- **Saturated Fat**: 1 g
- **Sodium**: 400 mg
- **Potassium**: 300 mg
- **Fiber**: 2 g
- **Sugar**: 1 g

4.9 Greek Yogurt Parfait

Ingredients

- 1 cup plain Greek yogurt
- 1/2 cup fresh berries (such as strawberries, blueberries, raspberries)
- 1/3 cup granola
- 1 tablespoon honey (optional)

Directions

1. **Layer half of the Greek yogurt** in the bottom of a parfait glass or mason jar.
2. **Top with half of the berries** and half of the granola.
3. **Repeat the layers** with the remaining yogurt, berries, and granola.
4. **If desired, drizzle honey** over the top layer.
5. **Serve immediately** or refrigerate until ready to serve.

Cooking and Prep Time

- **Prep Time**: 5 minutes
- **Total Time**: 5 minutes

Servings

This recipe makes approximately 1 serving.

Nutritional Information (per serving)

- **Calories**: 300 kcal
- **Protein**: 20 g
- **Carbohydrates**: 35 g
- **Fat**: 8 g
- **Saturated Fat**: 2 g
- **Sodium**: 100 mg
- **Potassium**: 300 mg
- **Fiber**: 5 g
- **Sugar**: 20 g

4.10 Cinnamon Quinoa

Ingredients

- 1 cup quinoa
- 2 cups water or almond milk (for added creaminess)
- 1 teaspoon ground cinnamon
- 2 tablespoons maple syrup (or honey, optional)
- 1/4 teaspoon salt
- 1/2 cup raisins or dried cranberries (optional)
- 1/4 cup chopped nuts (such as walnuts or almonds, optional)
- Fresh fruit for topping (such as banana slices or berries, optional)

Directions

1. **Rinse the Quinoa**: Place the quinoa in a fine mesh strainer and rinse under cold running water for a few minutes to remove any bitterness.
2. **Cook the Quinoa**: In a medium saucepan, combine the rinsed quinoa, water or almond milk, cinnamon, and salt. Bring to a boil over medium-high heat.
3. **Simmer**: Once boiling, reduce the heat to low, cover, and simmer for about 15 minutes, or until the quinoa is fluffy and has absorbed the liquid. Remove from heat and let it sit, covered, for 5 minutes.
4. **Add Sweetener and Mix**: Fluff the quinoa with a fork and stir in the maple syrup (if using), raisins or dried cranberries, and chopped nuts.
5. **Serve**: Serve warm, topped with fresh fruit if desired.

Cooking and Prep Time

- **Prep Time**: 5 minutes
- **Cook Time**: 20 minutes
- **Total Time**: 25 minutes

Servings

This recipe makes approximately 4 servings.

Nutritional Information (per serving)

- **Calories**: 180 kcal
- **Protein**: 6 g
- **Carbohydrates**: 32 g
- **Fat**: 4 g
- **Saturated Fat**: 0.5 g
- **Sodium**: 50 mg
- **Potassium**: 250 mg
- **Fiber**: 3 g
- **Sugar**: 4 g (without added sweetener)

4.11 Sweet Potato Hash

Ingredients

- 2 lb (900 g) sweet potatoes, peeled and cut into 1/2-inch pieces
- 1/4 cup (60 mL) low-sodium vegetable broth
- 3 garlic cloves, minced
- 1 small onion, chopped
- 1 small red bell pepper, chopped
- 1 small green bell pepper, chopped
- 1 tablespoon (15 mL) sweet paprika
- Salt and pepper (to taste)

Directions

1. **Prepare the Sweet Potatoes**: Place the sweet potatoes in a large saucepan and cover with water. Simmer for about 15 to 17 minutes until tender. Drain and set aside.
2. **Sauté the Vegetables**: In a large skillet, heat the vegetable broth over medium heat. Add the minced garlic, chopped onion, and bell peppers. Cook for about 4 minutes until the vegetables are softened.
3. **Season and Combine**: Add the sweet paprika, salt, and black pepper to the skillet. Stir to combine and continue cooking for another 5 minutes until the vegetables are soft.
4. **Mix in Sweet Potatoes**: Add the cooked sweet potatoes to the skillet and stir to heat through. Adjust seasoning with additional salt or pepper if needed.
5. **Serve**: Serve warm as a side dish or as a base for eggs or avocado.

Cooking and Prep Time

- **Prep Time**: 10 minutes
- **Cook Time**: 25 minutes
- **Total Time**: 35 minutes

Servings

This recipe makes approximately 4 servings.

Nutritional Information (per serving)

- **Calories**: 198 kcal
- **Protein**: 4 g
- **Carbohydrates**: 46 g
- **Fat**: 0.7 g
- **Saturated Fat**: 0.1 g
- **Cholesterol**: 0 mg
- **Sodium**: 105 mg
- **Fiber**: 7 g
- **Sugar**: 15 g
- **Vitamin A**: 22,197 mcg (from sweet potatoes)

4.12 Mango Chia Pudding

Ingredients

- 1 cup coconut milk (or almond milk)
- 1/4 cup chia seeds
- 2 tablespoons maple syrup (or honey, to taste)
- 1 cup ripe mango, diced (fresh or frozen)
- 1/2 teaspoon vanilla extract (optional)
- Pinch of salt

Directions

1. **Mix the Chia Pudding**: In a medium bowl, whisk together the coconut milk, chia seeds, maple syrup, vanilla extract (if using), and a pinch of salt. Stir well to combine.
2. **Refrigerate**: Cover the bowl and refrigerate for at least 4 hours or overnight. This allows the chia seeds to absorb the liquid and thicken into a pudding-like consistency.
3. **Prepare the Mango**: If using fresh mango, peel and dice it into small pieces. If using frozen mango, allow it to thaw and then chop.
4. **Assemble the Pudding**: Once the chia pudding has set, give it a good stir. Layer the chia pudding in serving glasses or bowls, alternating with layers of diced mango.
5. **Serve**: Enjoy immediately or refrigerate until ready to serve. You can also top it with additional mango, nuts, or coconut flakes for extra flavor and texture.

Cooking and Prep Time

- **Prep Time**: 10 minutes
- **Chilling Time**: 4 hours (or overnight)
- **Total Time**: 4 hours 10 minutes (or overnight)

Servings

This recipe makes approximately 2 servings.

Nutritional Information (per serving)

- **Calories**: 250 kcal
- **Protein**: 5 g
- **Carbohydrates**: 36 g
- **Fat**: 12 g
- **Saturated Fat**: 10 g
- **Sodium**: 50 mg
- **Potassium**: 300 mg
- **Fiber**: 10 g
- **Sugar**: 8 g

4.13 Cottage Cheese and Peaches

Ingredients

- **1 cup cottage cheese** (low-fat or full-fat)
- **1 medium ripe peach**, sliced (fresh or canned in juice)
- **1 tablespoon honey** (optional, for sweetness)
- **1/4 teaspoon cinnamon** (optional, for flavor)
- **Chopped nuts** (such as almonds or walnuts, optional for crunch)
- **Mint leaves** (for garnish, optional)

Directions

1. **Prepare the Peaches**: If using fresh peaches, wash, peel (if desired), and slice them. If using canned peaches, drain them well.
2. **Combine Ingredients**: In a bowl, add the cottage cheese. Top it with the sliced peaches.
3. **Add Sweetener and Spice**: Drizzle honey over the top if you prefer added sweetness. Sprinkle cinnamon for extra flavor.
4. **Add Nuts**: If using, sprinkle chopped nuts on top for added texture and nutrition.
5. **Garnish and Serve**: Garnish with fresh mint leaves if desired. Serve immediately and enjoy!

Cooking and Prep Time

- **Prep Time**: 5 minutes
- **Total Time**: 5 minutes

Servings

This recipe serves 1-2, depending on portion size.

Nutritional Information (per serving)

- **Calories**: 200 kcal
- **Protein**: 20 g

- **Carbohydrates**: 25 g
- **Fat**: 5 g
- **Saturated Fat**: 2 g
- **Sodium**: 350 mg
- **Potassium**: 400 mg
- **Fiber**: 2 g
- **Sugar**: 10 g (varies with honey and peach type)

4.14 Spinach and Feta Wrap

Ingredients

- 4 large whole wheat tortillas
- 2 cups fresh spinach, chopped
- 4 ounces feta cheese, crumbled
- 1 small onion, finely chopped
- 1 red bell pepper, diced
- 2 cloves garlic, minced
- 1 tablespoon olive oil
- Salt and pepper (to taste)
- 1 teaspoon dried oregano (optional)
- 1/2 teaspoon red pepper flakes (optional, for heat)

Directions

1. **Sauté the Vegetables**: In a large skillet, heat the olive oil over medium heat. Add the chopped onion and bell pepper, and sauté for about 5 minutes until softened. Add the minced garlic and cook for an additional minute until fragrant.
2. **Add Spinach**: Stir in the chopped spinach and cook until wilted, about 2-3 minutes. Season with salt, pepper, and oregano (if using).
3. **Mix in Feta**: Remove the skillet from heat and gently fold in the crumbled feta cheese.
4. **Assemble the Wraps**: Lay out the tortillas on a clean surface. Divide the spinach and feta mixture evenly among the tortillas, placing it in the center of each.
5. **Wrap It Up**: Fold in the sides of the tortilla, then roll it up tightly from the bottom to the top.
6. **Serve**: You can serve the wraps as is, or grill them in the skillet for 2-3 minutes on each side until golden brown and crispy.

Cooking and Prep Time

- **Prep Time**: 10 minutes
- **Cook Time**: 10 minutes
- **Total Time**: 20 minutes

Servings

This recipe makes approximately 4 servings.

Nutritional Information (per serving)

- **Calories**: 220 kcal
- **Protein**: 8 g
- **Carbohydrates**: 30 g
- **Fat**: 8 g
- **Saturated Fat**: 3 g
- **Sodium**: 400 mg
- **Potassium**: 300 mg
- **Fiber**: 4 g
- **Sugar**: 2 g

Chapter 4: Lunch Recipes

5.1 Quinoa and Vegetable Salad

Ingredients

- 1 cup quinoa, rinsed and drained
- 2 cups vegetable broth (or water)
- 1 bell pepper, diced (any color)
- 1 cucumber, diced
- 1 cup cherry tomatoes, halved
- 1/2 red onion, finely chopped
- 1 cup corn (fresh, frozen, or canned)
- 1/4 cup fresh parsley, chopped
- 1/4 cup olive oil
- 2 tablespoons lemon juice
- 1 teaspoon garlic powder
- Salt and pepper (to taste)

Directions

1. **Cook the Quinoa**: In a medium saucepan, combine the quinoa and vegetable broth (or water). Bring to a boil over medium-high heat. Once boiling, reduce the heat to low, cover, and let it simmer for about 15 minutes, or until the liquid is absorbed. Remove from heat and let it sit covered for 5 minutes. Fluff with a fork.
2. **Prepare the Vegetables**: While the quinoa is cooking, chop the bell pepper, cucumber, cherry tomatoes, red onion, and parsley.
3. **Combine Ingredients**: In a large bowl, combine the cooked quinoa, diced vegetables, corn, and parsley.
4. **Make the Dressing**: In a small bowl, whisk together the olive oil, lemon juice, garlic powder, salt, and pepper.

5. **Dress the Salad**: Pour the dressing over the quinoa and vegetable mixture. Toss gently to combine, ensuring all ingredients are well coated.
6. **Serve**: Serve immediately or refrigerate for 30 minutes to allow the flavors to meld. This salad can be enjoyed cold or at room temperature.

Cooking and Prep Time

- **Prep Time**: 15 minutes
- **Cook Time**: 20 minutes
- **Total Time**: 35 minutes

Servings

This recipe makes approximately 4 servings.

Nutritional Information (per serving)

- **Calories**: 220 kcal
- **Protein**: 6 g
- **Carbohydrates**: 30 g
- **Fat**: 10 g
- **Saturated Fat**: 1.5 g
- **Sodium**: 200 mg
- **Potassium**: 400 mg
- **Fiber**: 5 g
- **Sugar**: 2 g

5.2 Grilled Chicken Wraps

Ingredients

- 1 lb boneless, skinless chicken breasts
- 4 whole wheat tortillas (or your choice of wrap)
- 1 cup shredded romaine lettuce
- 1 cup diced tomatoes
- 1/2 cup sliced cucumber
- 1/4 cup crumbled feta cheese

For the Marinade:

- 2 tablespoons olive oil
- 2 tablespoons lemon juice
- 1 teaspoon dried oregano
- 1/2 teaspoon garlic powder
- Salt and pepper (to taste)

For the Sauce:

- 1/4 cup plain Greek yogurt
- 1 tablespoon lemon juice
- 1 tablespoon chopped fresh parsley
- 1/4 teaspoon garlic powder
- Salt and pepper (to taste)

Directions

1. **Prepare the Marinade**: In a shallow dish, whisk together the olive oil, lemon juice, oregano, garlic powder, salt, and pepper.
2. **Add the Chicken**: Add the chicken breasts to the marinade, turning to coat both sides. Cover and refrigerate for at least 30 minutes, up to 4 hours.

3. **Grill the Chicken**: Preheat your grill to medium-high heat. Grill the chicken for 5-7 minutes per side, or until cooked through. Let it rest for 5 minutes, then slice or chop into bite-sized pieces.
4. **Make the Sauce**: In a small bowl, mix together the Greek yogurt, lemon juice, parsley, garlic powder, salt, and pepper.
5. **Assemble the Wraps**: Lay the tortillas on a flat surface. Divide the grilled chicken, romaine lettuce, tomatoes, and cucumber evenly among the tortillas. Drizzle the yogurt sauce over the top and sprinkle with feta cheese.
6. **Roll Up**: Fold the bottom of the tortilla over the filling, then fold in the sides and continue rolling tightly into a wrap.
7. **Serve**: Serve immediately or wrap in foil or parchment paper to enjoy on the go.

Cooking and Prep Time

- **Prep Time**: 15 minutes
- **Cook Time**: 10-15 minutes
- **Total Time**: 25-30 minutes

Servings

This recipe makes approximately 4 wraps.

Nutritional Information (per wrap)

- **Calories**: 350
- **Protein**: 32g
- **Carbohydrates**: 35g
- **Fat**: 10g
- **Saturated Fat**: 3g
- **Sodium**: 550mg
- **Fiber**: 5g
- **Sugar**: 2g

5.3 Lentil Soup

Ingredients

- ¼ cup extra virgin olive oil
- 1 medium yellow or white onion, chopped
- 2 carrots, peeled and chopped
- 4 garlic cloves, minced
- 2 teaspoons ground cumin
- 1 teaspoon curry powder
- ½ teaspoon dried thyme
- 1 large can (28 ounces) diced tomatoes, lightly drained
- 1 cup brown or green lentils, rinsed
- 4 cups vegetable broth
- 2 cups water
- 1 teaspoon salt (more to taste)
- Pinch of red pepper flakes (optional)
- Freshly ground black pepper, to taste
- 1 cup chopped fresh collard greens or kale
- 1 to 2 tablespoons lemon juice (to taste)

Directions

1. **Sauté the Vegetables**: In a large pot or Dutch oven, heat the olive oil over medium heat. Add the chopped onion and carrots, cooking until the onion is translucent, about 5 minutes.
2. **Add Garlic and Spices**: Stir in the minced garlic, cumin, curry powder, and thyme. Cook for an additional 30 seconds until fragrant.
3. **Incorporate Tomatoes and Lentils**: Add the drained diced tomatoes and stir to combine. Then, add the rinsed lentils, vegetable broth, water, salt, and red pepper flakes (if using). Bring the mixture to a boil.

4. **Simmer the Soup**: Once boiling, reduce the heat to maintain a gentle simmer. Cover partially and cook for about 25-30 minutes, or until the lentils are tender but still hold their shape.
5. **Blend the Soup (Optional)**: For a creamier texture, transfer 2 cups of the soup to a blender and purée until smooth. Return the puréed soup to the pot, or use an immersion blender to blend part of the soup directly in the pot.
6. **Add Greens and Final Seasoning**: Stir in the chopped greens and cook for an additional 5 minutes, or until the greens are tender. Remove from heat and stir in lemon juice. Adjust seasoning with salt, pepper, and more lemon juice to taste.
7. **Serve**: Ladle the soup into bowls and serve hot. Leftovers can be stored in the refrigerator for up to 4 days or frozen for several months.

Cooking and Prep Time

- **Prep Time**: 10 minutes
- **Cook Time**: 45 minutes
- **Total Time**: 55 minutes

Servings

This recipe yields approximately 4 servings.

Nutritional Information (per serving)

- **Calories**: 320 kcal
- **Protein**: 18 g
- **Carbohydrates**: 45 g
- **Fat**: 10 g
- **Saturated Fat**: 1.5 g
- **Sodium**: 600 mg
- **Potassium**: 600 mg
- **Fiber**: 15 g
- **Sugar**: 5 g

5.4 Stuffed Bell Peppers

Ingredients

- 4 large bell peppers (any color)
- 1 lb ground beef (or turkey, chicken, or a plant-based alternative)
- 1 cup cooked rice (white or brown)
- 1 small onion, chopped
- 2 cloves garlic, minced
- 1 can (14.5 oz) diced tomatoes (with juices)
- 1 teaspoon Italian seasoning
- 1 teaspoon salt
- 1/2 teaspoon black pepper
- 1 cup shredded cheese (cheddar, mozzarella, or your choice)
- 1 tablespoon olive oil
- Fresh parsley (for garnish, optional)

Directions

1. **Preheat the Oven**: Preheat your oven to 375°F (190°C).
2. **Prepare the Peppers**: Cut the tops off the bell peppers and remove the seeds and membranes. Place them upright in a baking dish.
3. **Cook the Filling**: In a large skillet, heat olive oil over medium heat. Add the chopped onion and garlic, sautéing until the onion is translucent (about 3-4 minutes). Add the ground meat and cook until browned, breaking it apart with a spoon.
4. **Add Other Ingredients**: Stir in the cooked rice, diced tomatoes (with their juices), Italian seasoning, salt, and pepper. Cook for an additional 2-3 minutes until heated through.
5. **Stuff the Peppers**: Spoon the filling into each bell pepper, packing it down gently. Top each stuffed pepper with shredded cheese.

6. **Bake**: Cover the baking dish with aluminum foil and bake in the preheated oven for 25 minutes. Remove the foil and bake for an additional 10-15 minutes, or until the peppers are tender and the cheese is bubbly and golden.
7. **Serve**: Remove from the oven and let cool slightly. Garnish with fresh parsley if desired. Serve warm.

Cooking and Prep Time

- **Prep Time**: 15 minutes
- **Cook Time**: 40 minutes
- **Total Time**: 55 minutes

Servings

This recipe serves approximately 4 servings (1 stuffed pepper per serving).

Nutritional Information (per serving)

- **Calories**: 320 kcal
- **Protein**: 24 g
- **Carbohydrates**: 30 g
- **Fat**: 14 g
- **Saturated Fat**: 7 g
- **Cholesterol**: 70 mg
- **Sodium**: 600 mg
- **Potassium**: 600 mg
- **Fiber**: 4 g
- **Sugar**: 5 g

5.5 Tuna Salad

Ingredients

- 2 (5-ounce) cans of tuna in water, drained
- 1/4 cup mayonnaise
- 1/4 cup plain Greek yogurt (optional for creaminess)
- 1/3 cup diced celery (about 1 rib)
- 3 tablespoons diced red onion
- 2 tablespoons diced cornichon pickles (or dill pickles)
- Handful of baby spinach, thinly sliced (optional)
- Salt and pepper (to taste)
- 1 tablespoon lemon juice (optional, for brightness)

Directions

1. **Drain the Tuna**: Open the cans of tuna and drain the liquid thoroughly. Use a fork to flake the tuna into a mixing bowl.
2. **Combine Ingredients**: Add the mayonnaise, Greek yogurt (if using), diced celery, diced red onion, cornichon pickles, and baby spinach to the bowl with the tuna.
3. **Mix Well**: Stir all the ingredients together until well combined. Season with salt, pepper, and lemon juice to taste.
4. **Serve**: Tuna salad can be served in various ways:
    - On whole wheat bread for sandwiches
    - In lettuce cups for a low-carb option
    - On crackers as a snack
    - Stuffed in a pita pocket
    - On a bed of greens for a salad
5.
6. **Chill (Optional)**: If you prefer, refrigerate the tuna salad for about 30 minutes to allow the flavors to meld before serving.

Cooking and Prep Time

- **Prep Time**: 10 minutes
- **Total Time**: 10 minutes

Servings

This recipe makes approximately 4 servings.

Nutritional Information (per serving)

- **Calories**: 220 kcal
- **Protein**: 20 g
- **Carbohydrates**: 5 g
- **Fat**: 12 g
- **Saturated Fat**: 2 g
- **Cholesterol**: 40 mg
- **Sodium**: 400 mg
- **Potassium**: 300 mg
- **Fiber**: 1 g
- **Sugar**: 2 g

5.6 Chicken Caesar Salad

Ingredients

For the Salad:

- 2 large boneless, skinless chicken breasts
- 1 tablespoon olive oil
- Salt and pepper (to taste)
- 1 large head of romaine lettuce, chopped
- 1/2 cup grated Parmesan cheese
- 1 cup homemade or store-bought croutons

For the Caesar Dressing:

- 1/2 cup mayonnaise
- 1 clove garlic, minced
- 2 tablespoons lemon juice
- 1 teaspoon Dijon mustard
- 1 teaspoon Worcestershire sauce
- 2 anchovy fillets (optional, for authentic flavor)
- Salt and pepper (to taste)
- 1/4 cup grated Parmesan cheese

Directions

1. **Prepare the Chicken**: Preheat your grill or stovetop grill pan over medium-high heat. Rub the chicken breasts with olive oil, and season with salt and pepper. Grill the chicken for about 6-7 minutes per side, or until fully cooked and the internal temperature reaches 165°F (75°C). Remove from heat and let rest for 5 minutes before slicing.
2. **Make the Dressing**: In a bowl, whisk together the mayonnaise, minced garlic, lemon juice, Dijon mustard, Worcestershire sauce, and anchovies (if using). Stir

in the grated Parmesan cheese and season with salt and pepper to taste. Adjust the consistency with a little water if needed.
3. **Assemble the Salad**: In a large bowl, combine the chopped romaine lettuce, sliced grilled chicken, croutons, and grated Parmesan cheese. Drizzle the Caesar dressing over the top and toss gently to coat all ingredients evenly.
4. **Serve**: Divide the salad among plates or serve in a large bowl. Garnish with additional Parmesan cheese and freshly ground black pepper if desired.

Cooking and Prep Time

- **Prep Time**: 15 minutes
- **Cook Time**: 15 minutes
- **Total Time**: 30 minutes

Servings

This recipe serves approximately 4 servings.

Nutritional Information (per serving)

- **Calories**: 400 kcal
- **Protein**: 30 g
- **Carbohydrates**: 15 g
- **Fat**: 25 g
- **Saturated Fat**: 5 g
- **Cholesterol**: 90 mg
- **Sodium**: 600 mg
- **Potassium**: 600 mg
- **Fiber**: 2 g
- **Sugar**: 1 g

5.7 Vegetable Stir-Fry

Ingredients

- 2 tablespoons olive oil or sesame oil
- 3 cloves garlic, minced
- 1 tablespoon grated fresh ginger
- 1 cup broccoli florets
- 1 cup sliced mushrooms
- 1 red bell pepper, sliced
- 1 cup snow peas or snap peas
- 1 cup sliced carrots
- 1 cup bean sprouts
- 2 green onions, sliced

For the Sauce:

- 3 tablespoons soy sauce
- 2 tablespoons rice vinegar
- 1 tablespoon honey or brown sugar
- 1 teaspoon sesame oil
- 1/2 teaspoon red pepper flakes (optional)
- 1 tablespoon cornstarch

Directions

1. **Make the Sauce**: In a small bowl, whisk together the soy sauce, rice vinegar, honey, sesame oil, red pepper flakes (if using), and cornstarch. Set aside.
2. **Prepare the Vegetables**: Chop or slice the garlic, ginger, broccoli, mushrooms, bell pepper, snow peas, carrots, and green onions.
3. **Stir-Fry the Vegetables**: Heat the oil in a large skillet or wok over high heat. Add the garlic and ginger and cook for 30 seconds, stirring constantly, until fragrant.

4. **Add the broccoli, mushrooms, bell pepper, snow peas, and carrots.** Stir-fry for 2-3 minutes, until the vegetables are crisp-tender.
5. **Add the bean sprouts and green onions.** Stir-fry for an additional minute.
6. **Pour the sauce over the vegetables and stir to coat evenly.** Cook for 1-2 minutes, until the sauce thickens slightly.
7. **Remove from heat and serve immediately**, over rice or noodles if desired.

Cooking and Prep Time

- **Prep Time**: 10 minutes
- **Cook Time**: 10 minutes
- **Total Time**: 20 minutes

Servings

This recipe serves approximately 4 people.

Nutritional Information (per serving)

- **Calories**: 150 kcal
- **Protein**: 5 g
- **Carbohydrates**: 20 g
- **Fat**: 7 g
- **Saturated Fat**: 1 g
- **Sodium**: 600 mg
- **Fiber**: 5 g
- **Sugar**: 8 g

5.8 Turkey and Avocado Sandwich

Ingredients

- 2 slices whole grain or sourdough bread
- 4 ounces sliced turkey breast (deli-style or leftover roasted turkey)
- 1/2 ripe avocado, sliced
- 1/2 cup fresh spinach or lettuce
- 1 medium tomato, sliced
- 1/4 small red onion, thinly sliced (optional)
- 1 tablespoon mayonnaise (or Greek yogurt for a healthier option)
- Salt and pepper (to taste)
- 1 teaspoon lemon juice (optional, to prevent avocado from browning)

Directions

1. **Prepare the Avocado**: In a small bowl, mash the avocado with a fork. If desired, add lemon juice, salt, and pepper to taste.
2. **Toast the Bread**: Lightly toast the slices of bread until golden brown.
3. **Assemble the Sandwich**: Spread mayonnaise (or Greek yogurt) on one slice of the toasted bread. Layer the spinach or lettuce, sliced turkey, avocado, tomato, and red onion (if using) on top.
4. **Season**: Sprinkle a little salt and pepper over the vegetables for added flavor.
5. **Top and Serve**: Place the second slice of bread on top, cut the sandwich in half if desired, and serve immediately.

Cooking and Prep Time

- **Prep Time**: 10 minutes
- **Cook Time**: 2-3 minutes (for toasting)
- **Total Time**: 12-13 minutes

Servings

This recipe serves 1 sandwich.

Nutritional Information (per sandwich)

- **Calories**: 350 kcal
- **Protein**: 25 g
- **Carbohydrates**: 30 g
- **Fat**: 15 g
- **Saturated Fat**: 2 g
- **Sodium**: 600 mg
- **Potassium**: 800 mg
- **Fiber**: 8 g
- **Sugar**: 3 g

5.9 Tomato Basil Soup

Ingredients

- 2 tablespoons olive oil
- 1 medium onion, chopped
- 3 cloves garlic, minced
- 2 cans (14.5 oz each) diced tomatoes (or 4 cups fresh tomatoes, chopped)
- 1 cup vegetable broth (or chicken broth)
- 1 teaspoon sugar (optional, to balance acidity)
- 1/2 teaspoon salt (or to taste)
- 1/4 teaspoon black pepper
- 1/2 cup fresh basil leaves, chopped (plus extra for garnish)
- 1/2 cup heavy cream (or coconut milk for a dairy-free option)

Directions

1. **Sauté the Aromatics**: In a large pot, heat the olive oil over medium heat. Add the chopped onion and sauté until translucent, about 5 minutes. Stir in the minced garlic and cook for an additional minute until fragrant.
2. **Add Tomatoes and Broth**: Pour in the diced tomatoes (with their juices) and the vegetable broth. If using fresh tomatoes, add them at this stage. Stir to combine.
3. **Season the Soup**: Add sugar (if using), salt, and black pepper. Bring the mixture to a simmer and cook for about 15-20 minutes to allow the flavors to meld.
4. **Blend the Soup**: Using an immersion blender, blend the soup until smooth. Alternatively, you can carefully transfer the soup in batches to a blender to puree.
5. **Add Basil and Cream**: Stir in the chopped basil and heavy cream. Heat through for another 5 minutes, but do not bring to a boil.
6. **Serve**: Ladle the soup into bowls and garnish with additional fresh basil if desired. Serve hot with crusty bread or a grilled cheese sandwich.

Cooking and Prep Time

- **Prep Time**: 10 minutes
- **Cook Time**: 25 minutes
- **Total Time**: 35 minutes

Servings

This recipe serves approximately 4 servings.

Nutritional Information (per serving)

- **Calories**: 220 kcal
- **Protein**: 4 g
- **Carbohydrates**: 18 g
- **Fat**: 15 g
- **Saturated Fat**: 7 g
- **Cholesterol**: 40 mg
- **Sodium**: 500 mg
- **Potassium**: 400 mg
- **Fiber**: 3 g
- **Sugar**: 4 g

5.10 Spinach and Mushroom Quiche

Ingredients

- 2 tablespoons olive oil
- 1 medium onion, chopped
- 3 cloves garlic, minced
- 2 cans (14.5 oz each) diced tomatoes (or 4 cups fresh tomatoes, chopped)
- 1 cup vegetable broth (or chicken broth)
- 1 teaspoon sugar (optional, to balance acidity)
- 1/2 teaspoon salt (or to taste)
- 1/4 teaspoon black pepper
- 1/2 cup fresh basil leaves, chopped (plus extra for garnish)
- 1/2 cup heavy cream (or coconut milk for a dairy-free option)

Directions

1. **Sauté the Aromatics**: In a large pot, heat the olive oil over medium heat. Add the chopped onion and sauté until translucent, about 5 minutes. Stir in the minced garlic and cook for an additional minute until fragrant.
2. **Add Tomatoes and Broth**: Pour in the diced tomatoes (with their juices) and the vegetable broth. If using fresh tomatoes, add them at this stage. Stir to combine.
3. **Season the Soup**: Add sugar (if using), salt, and black pepper. Bring the mixture to a simmer and cook for about 15-20 minutes to allow the flavors to meld.
4. **Blend the Soup**: Using an immersion blender, blend the soup until smooth. Alternatively, you can carefully transfer the soup in batches to a blender to puree.
5. **Add Basil and Cream**: Stir in the chopped basil and heavy cream. Heat through for another 5 minutes, but do not bring to a boil.
6. **Serve**: Ladle the soup into bowls and garnish with additional fresh basil if desired. Serve hot with crusty bread or a grilled cheese sandwich.

Cooking and Prep Time

- **Prep Time**: 10 minutes
- **Cook Time**: 25 minutes
- **Total Time**: 35 minutes

Servings

This recipe serves approximately 4 servings.

Nutritional Information (per serving)

- **Calories**: 220 kcal
- **Protein**: 4 g
- **Carbohydrates**: 18 g
- **Fat**: 15 g
- **Saturated Fat**: 7 g
- **Cholesterol**: 40 mg
- **Sodium**: 500 mg
- **Potassium**: 400 mg
- **Fiber**: 3 g
- **Sugar**: 4 g

5.11 Couscous Salad

Ingredients

- 1 cup couscous
- 1 1/4 cups vegetable broth (or water)
- 1 cup cherry tomatoes, halved
- 1 cucumber, diced
- 1 bell pepper, diced (any color)
- 1/4 red onion, finely chopped
- 1/2 cup parsley, chopped
- 1/4 cup feta cheese, crumbled (optional)
- 1/4 cup olive oil
- 2 tablespoons lemon juice
- 1 teaspoon dried oregano
- Salt and pepper (to taste)

Directions

1. **Cook the Couscous**: In a medium saucepan, bring the vegetable broth (or water) to a boil. Stir in the couscous, cover, and remove from heat. Let it sit for about 5 minutes, or until the liquid is absorbed. Fluff with a fork and let it cool.
2. **Prepare the Vegetables**: While the couscous is cooling, chop the cherry tomatoes, cucumber, bell pepper, red onion, and parsley.
3. **Make the Dressing**: In a small bowl, whisk together the olive oil, lemon juice, dried oregano, salt, and pepper.
4. **Combine Ingredients**: In a large bowl, combine the cooled couscous, chopped vegetables, and feta cheese (if using). Pour the dressing over the salad and toss gently to combine.
5. **Serve**: Taste and adjust seasoning if necessary. Serve immediately or refrigerate for 30 minutes to allow the flavors to meld.

Cooking and Prep Time

- **Prep Time**: 10 minutes
- **Cook Time**: 5 minutes
- **Total Time**: 15 minutes

Servings

This recipe serves approximately 4 servings.

Nutritional Information (per serving)

- **Calories**: 220 kcal
- **Protein**: 6 g
- **Carbohydrates**: 30 g
- **Fat**: 10 g
- **Saturated Fat**: 1.5 g
- **Sodium**: 300 mg
- **Potassium**: 250 mg
- **Fiber**: 3 g
- **Sugar**: 2 g

5.12 Chicken and Rice Bowl

Ingredients

- 1 lb boneless, skinless chicken breasts, cut into bite-sized pieces
- 1 cup uncooked rice (white, brown, or jasmine)
- 2 cups chicken broth (or water)
- 2 tablespoons olive oil
- 1 teaspoon garlic powder
- 1 teaspoon onion powder
- 1 teaspoon paprika
- Salt and pepper (to taste)
- 1 cup mixed vegetables (such as bell peppers, broccoli, and carrots)
- 2 tablespoons soy sauce
- 1 tablespoon honey (or brown sugar)
- 1 tablespoon lemon juice (or lime juice)
- Chopped green onions (for garnish, optional)
- Sesame seeds (for garnish, optional)

Directions

1. **Cook the Rice**: In a medium saucepan, bring the chicken broth (or water) to a boil. Add the uncooked rice, reduce the heat to low, cover, and let it simmer for about 15-20 minutes (or according to package instructions) until the rice is cooked and the liquid is absorbed. Remove from heat and fluff with a fork.
2. **Prepare the Chicken**: While the rice is cooking, heat the olive oil in a large skillet over medium-high heat. Season the chicken pieces with garlic powder, onion powder, paprika, salt, and pepper.
3. **Cook the Chicken**: Add the seasoned chicken to the skillet and cook for about 5-7 minutes, stirring occasionally, until the chicken is browned and cooked through.

4. **Add Vegetables**: Stir in the mixed vegetables and cook for an additional 3-5 minutes, until the vegetables are tender.
5. **Make the Sauce**: In a small bowl, whisk together the soy sauce, honey, and lemon juice. Pour the sauce over the chicken and vegetables, stirring to coat evenly. Cook for another minute or two until heated through.
6. **Assemble the Bowls**: Divide the cooked rice among serving bowls. Top with the chicken and vegetable mixture.
7. **Garnish and Serve**: Garnish with chopped green onions and sesame seeds if desired. Serve warm.

Cooking and Prep Time

- **Prep Time**: 10 minutes
- **Cook Time**: 25 minutes
- **Total Time**: 35 minutes

Servings

This recipe serves approximately 4 servings.

Nutritional Information (per serving)

- **Calories**: 350 kcal
- **Protein**: 30 g
- **Carbohydrates**: 45 g
- **Fat**: 8 g
- **Saturated Fat**: 1.5 g
- **Cholesterol**: 70 mg
- **Sodium**: 600 mg
- **Potassium**: 600 mg
- **Fiber**: 3 g
- **Sugar**: 5 g

5.13 Veggie Burger

Ingredients

- 1 (15 oz) can black beans, drained and rinsed
- 1 cup cooked quinoa (or brown rice)
- 1 cup grated carrots
- 1/2 cup rolled oats
- 1/2 cup breadcrumbs
- 1/4 cup finely chopped onion
- 2 cloves garlic, minced
- 1 teaspoon cumin
- 1/2 teaspoon chili powder
- 1/4 teaspoon smoked paprika
- Salt and pepper (to taste)
- 1 tablespoon olive oil (for cooking)
- Whole wheat buns, lettuce, tomato, avocado (for serving)

Directions

1. In a large bowl, mash the black beans with a fork or potato masher, leaving some chunks.
2. Add the cooked quinoa, grated carrots, rolled oats, breadcrumbs, onion, garlic, cumin, chili powder, smoked paprika, salt, and pepper. Mix well until fully combined.
3. Divide the mixture into 6 equal portions and shape them into patties, about 1/2 inch thick.
4. In a large skillet, heat the olive oil over medium heat. Cook the veggie patties for 3-4 minutes per side, or until golden brown and crispy.
5. Serve the veggie burgers on whole wheat buns with your favorite toppings like lettuce, tomato, and avocado.

Cooking and Prep Time

- **Prep Time**: 15 minutes
- **Cook Time**: 8-10 minutes
- **Total Time**: 23-25 minutes

Servings

This recipe makes approximately 6 veggie burgers.

Nutritional Information (per burger, without bun and toppings)

- **Calories**: 200 kcal
- **Protein**: 8 g
- **Carbohydrates**: 30 g
- **Fat**: 5 g
- **Saturated Fat**: 1 g
- **Sodium**: 350 mg
- **Fiber**: 7 g
- **Sugar**: 2 g

5.14 Mediterranean Chickpea Salad

Ingredients

- 1 (15 oz) can chickpeas, drained and rinsed
- 1 cup cherry tomatoes, halved
- 1 cucumber, diced
- 1/2 red onion, finely chopped
- 1/2 cup roasted red peppers, diced
- 1/2 cup feta cheese, crumbled (optional)
- 1/4 cup parsley, chopped
- 1/4 cup kalamata olives, pitted and sliced (optional)

For the Dressing:

- 3 tablespoons olive oil
- 1 tablespoon red wine vinegar
- 1 teaspoon Dijon mustard
- 1 teaspoon dried oregano
- Salt and pepper (to taste)
- 1 small clove garlic, minced (optional)

Directions

1. **Prepare the Dressing**: In a small bowl, whisk together the olive oil, red wine vinegar, Dijon mustard, dried oregano, salt, pepper, and minced garlic until well combined. Set aside.
2. **Combine the Salad Ingredients**: In a large bowl, add the chickpeas, cherry tomatoes, cucumber, red onion, roasted red peppers, feta cheese (if using), parsley, and olives (if using).
3. **Dress the Salad**: Pour the dressing over the salad and toss gently to combine all ingredients evenly.

4. **Serve**: Taste and adjust seasoning if necessary. Serve immediately or refrigerate for 30 minutes to allow the flavors to meld.

Cooking and Prep Time

- **Prep Time**: 10 minutes
- **Total Time**: 10 minutes

Servings

This recipe serves approximately 4 servings.

Nutritional Information (per serving)

- **Calories**: 220 kcal
- **Protein**: 10 g
- **Carbohydrates**: 25 g
- **Fat**: 10 g
- **Saturated Fat**: 3 g
- **Sodium**: 400 mg
- **Potassium**: 400 mg
- **Fiber**: 6 g
- **Sugar**: 3 g

Chapter 5: Dinner Recipes

6.1 Baked Salmon with Herbs

Ingredients

- 1.5 lbs salmon fillet (skin on or off)
- 2 tbsp olive oil
- 1 tbsp minced garlic (about 3 cloves)
- 1-2 tbsp chopped fresh herbs (such as thyme, parsley, dill or rosemary)
- 1 tbsp lemon juice
- Salt and pepper to taste

Instructions

1. **Preheat oven** to 400°F. Line a rimmed baking sheet with foil and lightly grease or spray with non-stick cooking spray.
2. **Place salmon** skin-side down on the prepared baking sheet.
3. **In a small bowl**, combine olive oil, minced garlic, lemon juice, and chopped herbs. Mix well.
4. **Spread the herb mixture** evenly over the top of the salmon. Season with salt and pepper.
5. **Bake for 15-20 minutes**, until salmon is opaque and flakes easily with a fork. For a browned top, broil for 2 minutes at the end.
6. **Allow salmon to rest** for 5 minutes before serving. Transfer to a serving dish or cut into portions.

Prep Time: 5 minutes

Cook Time: 15-20 minutes

Total Time: 20-25 minutes

Serving Size: 4-6

Nutrition (per serving)

- Calories: 300
- Fat: 18g
- Carbs: 0g
- Protein: 34g
- Sodium: 120mg
- Potassium: 700mg
- Omega-3s: 2.5g

6.2 Turkey and Vegetable Stir-Fry

Ingredients

- 1 lb ground turkey
- 2 tablespoons olive oil (divided)
- 1 medium onion, diced
- 1 cup broccoli florets
- 1 red bell pepper, diced
- 1 cup carrots, sliced
- 1 zucchini, diced
- 3 cloves garlic, minced
- 1 tablespoon fresh ginger, minced
- 3 tablespoons low-sodium soy sauce
- 1 tablespoon hoisin sauce (optional)
- Salt and pepper to taste
- Optional toppings: sesame seeds, chopped scallions

Directions

1. **Prep the Ingredients**: Gather and prepare all the vegetables by washing and chopping them into bite-sized pieces.
2. **Cook the Turkey**: In a large skillet or wok, heat 1 tablespoon of olive oil over medium-high heat. Add the ground turkey and cook until browned and cooked through, about 5-7 minutes. Break it up with a spoon as it cooks. Once done, transfer the turkey to a plate and set aside.
3. **Sauté the Vegetables**: In the same skillet, add the remaining tablespoon of olive oil. Add the diced onion and sauté for about 2 minutes until softened. Then, add the garlic and ginger, cooking for an additional minute until fragrant.
4. **Add Remaining Vegetables**: Add the broccoli, bell pepper, carrots, and zucchini to the skillet. Stir-fry for about 5-7 minutes until the vegetables are tender-crisp.

5. **Combine and Season**: Return the cooked turkey to the skillet. Pour in the soy sauce and hoisin sauce (if using), stirring well to combine. Cook for another 2-3 minutes until everything is heated through. Season with salt and pepper to taste.
6. **Serve**: Serve the stir-fry hot, garnished with sesame seeds or chopped scallions if desired.

Cooking and Prep Time

- **Prep Time**: 10 minutes
- **Cook Time**: 15 minutes
- **Total Time**: 25 minutes

Serving Size

- Serves: 4

Nutrition (per serving)

- Calories: 280
- Protein: 28g
- Carbohydrates: 12g
- Fat: 14g
- Fiber: 3g
- Sodium: 500mg

6.3 Spaghetti Squash with Marinara

Ingredients

- 1 medium spaghetti squash (about 2-3 lbs)
- 1 tablespoon olive oil
- 1 (28oz) can whole peeled tomatoes
- 8 cloves garlic, peeled and thinly sliced
- 1 teaspoon dried oregano
- 1/4 cup fresh basil, chopped
- Salt and pepper to taste
- Parmesan cheese for serving (optional)

Instructions

1. **Preheat oven** to 400°F. Cut the spaghetti squash in half lengthwise and scoop out the seeds. Place cut-side down on a rimmed baking sheet. Roast for 40-50 minutes until tender when pierced with a fork.
2. **Meanwhile, make the marinara sauce**. In a large skillet, heat the olive oil over medium heat. Add the garlic and cook for 1 minute until fragrant.
3. **Add the canned tomatoes** and their juices, crushing them with your hands as you add them to the pan. Stir in the oregano and season with salt and pepper.
4. **Simmer the sauce for 15-20 minutes**, stirring occasionally, until thickened. Remove from heat and stir in the fresh basil.
5. **When the squash is done**, let it cool slightly. Use a fork to scrape the flesh into long strands, creating "spaghetti".
6. **Add the spaghetti squash strands** to the marinara sauce and toss to coat.
7. **Serve immediately**, garnished with Parmesan cheese if desired. Enjoy!

Prep Time: 10 minutes

Cook Time: 40-50 minutes

Total Time: 50-60 minutes

Servings: 4

Nutrition (per serving)

- Calories: 175
- Total Fat: 7g
- Saturated Fat: 1g
- Cholesterol: 0mg
- Sodium: 680mg
- Total Carbs: 27g
- Dietary Fiber: 5g
- Total Sugars: 10g
- Protein: 5g

6.4 Beef and Broccoli

Ingredients

- **For the Beef:**
    - 1 lb flank steak, very thinly sliced into bite-sized strips
    - 2 tablespoons olive oil (or vegetable oil), divided
    - 1 lb broccoli, cut into florets (about 6 cups)
- **For the Stir Fry Sauce:**
    - 1 teaspoon fresh ginger, grated
    - 2 teaspoons garlic, grated (from about 3 cloves)
    - 1/2 cup hot water
    - 6 tablespoons low-sodium soy sauce (or gluten-free Tamari)
    - 3 tablespoons packed light brown sugar
    - 1 1/2 tablespoons cornstarch
    - 1/4 teaspoon black pepper
    - 2 tablespoons sesame oil

Instructions

1. **Prep the Ingredients:**
    - Start by slicing the flank steak against the grain into thin strips. Cut the broccoli into small florets.
2. **Make the Sauce:**
    - In a bowl, combine the soy sauce, hot water, brown sugar, cornstarch, ginger, garlic, black pepper, and sesame oil. Stir well to dissolve the sugar and cornstarch, and set aside.
3. **Cook the Broccoli:**
    - Heat 1 tablespoon of oil in a large skillet over medium heat. Add the broccoli florets and sauté for about 4-5 minutes until they are bright green and tender-crisp. Remove the broccoli from the skillet and set aside.

4. **Cook the Beef:**
   - Increase the heat to high and add the remaining tablespoon of oil. Add the sliced beef in a single layer and sauté for about 2 minutes on each side until cooked through.
5. **Combine and Thicken the Sauce:**
   - Pour the prepared sauce over the beef, reduce the heat to medium-low, and let it simmer for about 3-4 minutes until the sauce thickens. Return the broccoli to the skillet and stir to combine.
6. **Serve:**
   - Serve hot over cooked white rice or brown rice, if desired. Garnish with sesame seeds if you like.

Cooking and Prep Time

- **Prep Time:** 15 minutes
- **Cook Time:** 15 minutes
- **Total Time:** 30 minutes
- **Servings:** 4

Nutrition (per serving)

- **Calories:** Approximately 300
- **Total Fat:** 12g
- **Saturated Fat:** 2g
- **Cholesterol:** 70mg
- **Sodium:** 800mg
- **Total Carbohydrates:** 25g
- **Dietary Fiber:** 4g
- **Total Sugars:** 5g
- **Protein:** 25g

6.5 Chicken Alfredo with Zoodles

Ingredients

- 3 medium zucchinis, spiralized into noodles
- 1 lb boneless, skinless chicken breasts, thinly sliced
- 2 tbsp olive oil, divided
- 1 tsp Italian seasoning
- 1/2 tsp garlic powder
- Salt and pepper to taste
- 2 cloves garlic, minced
- 3/4 cup heavy cream
- 1/2 cup grated parmesan cheese, plus more for serving
- 2 tbsp chopped fresh parsley, plus more for serving

Instructions

1. **Season the chicken** with Italian seasoning, garlic powder, salt and pepper.
2. **Heat 1 tbsp olive oil** in a large skillet over medium-high heat. Add the chicken and cook for 3-5 minutes per side until cooked through. Remove chicken from skillet and set aside.
3. **In the same skillet**, heat the remaining 1 tbsp olive oil over medium heat. Add the minced garlic and cook for 1 minute until fragrant.
4. **Add the spiralized zucchini noodles** to the skillet. Cook for 3-4 minutes, stirring occasionally, until zucchini is just tender but still has a bite.
5. **Pour in the heavy cream** and parmesan cheese. Stir to combine and cook for 2-3 minutes until sauce thickens slightly.
6. **Add the cooked chicken** back to the skillet and toss everything together.
7. **Remove from heat** and stir in the chopped parsley. Season with salt and pepper to taste.
8. **Serve immediately**, garnished with extra parmesan and parsley if desired.

Prep Time: 10 minutes

Cook Time: 15 minutes

Total Time: 25 minutes

Servings: 4

Nutrition (per serving)

- Calories: 420
- Total Fat: 28g
- Saturated Fat: 13g
- Cholesterol: 135mg
- Sodium: 480mg
- Total Carbs: 10g
- Dietary Fiber: 3g
- Total Sugars: 4g
- Protein: 38g

6.6 Grilled Shrimp Tacos

Ingredients

- **For the Shrimp:**
    - 1 lb shrimp, peeled and deveined
    - 1 tbsp olive oil
    - 1 tbsp chipotle powder
    - 1 tbsp onion powder
    - 1 tbsp fine sea salt
    - 2 limes, halved
- **For the Tacos:**
    - ½ cup red cabbage, chopped
    - ½ cup white onion, diced
    - ¼ cup fresh cilantro, chopped
    - Corn tortillas
    - Sliced avocado (optional)
    - Sour cream (optional)

Directions

1. **Prepare the Shrimp:**
    - In a bowl, combine the shrimp with olive oil, chipotle powder, onion powder, and fine sea salt. Squeeze the juice of one lime over the shrimp and mix well.
2. **Preheat the Grill:**
    - Prepare your grill for direct heat and preheat to medium-high (about 375-400°F). If using charcoal, let it burn until the coals are white hot.
3. **Grill the Shrimp:**
    - Place the shrimp on the grill and cook for about 2 minutes on each side, or until they turn pink and are no longer translucent. Remove from the grill.

4. **Warm the Tortillas:**
    - Place corn tortillas on the grill for about 30 seconds per side to warm them up. For extra texture, stack two tortillas together while grilling.
5. **Assemble the Tacos:**
    - On each tortilla, layer the grilled shrimp, followed by red cabbage, diced onion, fresh cilantro, and sliced avocado if desired. Add a dollop of sour cream and a squeeze of lime juice for additional flavor.
6. **Serve:**
    - Serve the tacos immediately with lime wedges on the side.

Cooking and Prep Time

- **Prep Time:** 15 minutes
- **Cook Time:** 5 minutes
- **Total Time:** 20 minutes
- **Servings:** 4

Nutrition (per serving)

- **Calories:** Approximately 250
- **Total Fat:** 10g
- **Saturated Fat:** 1.5g
- **Cholesterol:** 150mg
- **Sodium:** 800mg
- **Total Carbohydrates:** 20g
- **Dietary Fiber:** 3g
- **Total Sugars:** 2g
- **Protein:** 20g

6.7 Quinoa Stuffed Peppers

Ingredients

- 6 medium bell peppers (any color)
- 1 cup uncooked quinoa, rinsed and drained
- 2 cups vegetable broth
- 1 tablespoon olive oil
- 1 small onion, chopped
- 2 garlic cloves, minced
- 1 (15 oz) can diced tomatoes
- 1 (15 oz) can black beans, rinsed and drained
- 1 cup frozen corn, thawed
- 1 teaspoon cumin
- 1 teaspoon paprika
- ½ teaspoon salt
- ¼ teaspoon black pepper
- 1 cup shredded Monterey Jack cheese (or cheese of choice)
- Optional toppings: chopped fresh cilantro, diced avocado, sour cream

Instructions

1. Cook the quinoa in vegetable broth according to package instructions. Set aside.
2. Preheat oven to 375°F (190°C). Cut the tops off the bell peppers and remove seeds and membranes. Place peppers cut-side up in a baking dish and pour a small amount of water around them.
3. In a skillet, sauté the onion in olive oil over medium heat until softened, about 2-3 minutes. Add garlic and cook for 1 minute.
4. Stir in the cooked quinoa, diced tomatoes, black beans, corn, cumin, paprika, salt and pepper. Cook for 5 minutes.
5. Spoon the quinoa mixture into each bell pepper, packing it down slightly. Top with shredded cheese.

6. Cover baking dish with foil and bake for 25 minutes. Remove foil and bake 10-15 minutes more, until peppers are tender and cheese is melted.
7. Remove from oven and let cool slightly. Garnish with optional toppings like cilantro, avocado or sour cream if desired. Serve hot.

Cooking and Prep Time

- **Prep Time:** 15 minutes
- **Cook Time:** 40 minutes
- **Total Time:** 55 minutes
- **Servings:** 6

Nutrition (per serving)

- **Calories:** Approximately 286
- **Total Fat:** 9g
- **Saturated Fat:** 3g
- **Cholesterol:** 15mg
- **Sodium:** 600mg
- **Total Carbohydrates:** 39g
- **Dietary Fiber:** 9g
- **Total Sugars:** 3g
- **Protein:** 12g

6.8 Lemon Herb Chicken

Ingredients

- **For the Marinade:**
    - 2 tablespoons lemon zest
    - 1/3 cup fresh lemon juice
    - 2 cloves garlic, minced
    - 1 teaspoon dried basil (or 1 tablespoon fresh basil)
    - 1 teaspoon dried thyme (or 1 tablespoon fresh thyme)
    - 1 teaspoon dried rosemary (or 1 tablespoon fresh rosemary)
    - 1 teaspoon salt
    - 1 teaspoon pepper
    - 2 tablespoons olive oil
- **For the Chicken:**
    - 4-6 boneless, skinless chicken breasts

Directions

1. **Prepare the Marinade:**
    - In a zippered plastic bag or bowl, mix together the lemon zest, lemon juice, minced garlic, basil, thyme, rosemary, salt, pepper, and olive oil.
2. **Marinate the Chicken:**
    - Add the chicken breasts to the marinade, ensuring they are well coated.
    - Seal the bag or cover the bowl and refrigerate for 2-4 hours. Avoid marinating for longer than 4 hours to prevent the chicken from becoming mushy due to the acidity of the lemon juice.
3. **Preheat the Cooking Method:**
    - If grilling, preheat the grill to medium-high heat (about 375°F).
    - If baking, preheat the oven to 425°F.

4. **Cook the Chicken:**
    - **Grilling:** Remove the chicken from the marinade and grill for about 5-7 minutes on each side, or until the internal temperature reaches 165°F.
    - **Baking:** Place the marinated chicken breasts in a baking dish and bake for about 20-25 minutes, turning halfway through, until fully cooked.
5. **Serve:**
    - Let the chicken rest for a few minutes before slicing. Serve with your choice of sides, such as roasted vegetables or a fresh salad.

Cooking and Prep Time

- **Prep Time:** 15 minutes (plus marinating time)
- **Cook Time:** 20-25 minutes (grilling or baking)
- **Total Time:** Approximately 2 hours (including marinating)
- **Servings:** 4-6

Nutrition (per serving)

- **Calories:** Approximately 230
- **Total Fat:** 10g
- **Saturated Fat:** 1.5g
- **Cholesterol:** 75mg
- **Sodium:** 600mg
- **Total Carbohydrates:** 3g
- **Dietary Fiber:** 0g
- **Total Sugars:** 1g
- **Protein:** 30g

6.9 Vegetable Lasagna

Ingredients

- **For the Lasagna:**
    - 9-12 lasagna noodles (regular or no-boil)
    - 2 tablespoons olive oil
    - 1 medium onion, chopped
    - 3 cloves garlic, minced
    - 1 zucchini, diced
    - 1 bell pepper, diced
    - 1 cup mushrooms, sliced
    - 2 cups fresh spinach
    - 1 (24 oz) jar marinara sauce
    - 1 teaspoon dried oregano
    - 1 teaspoon dried basil
    - Salt and pepper to taste
- **For the Cheese Mixture:**
    - 15 oz ricotta cheese
    - 1 cup grated Parmesan cheese
    - 1 cup shredded mozzarella cheese (plus more for topping)
    - 1 egg
    - 1 tablespoon fresh parsley, chopped (optional)

Directions

1. **Preheat the Oven:**
    - Preheat your oven to 375°F (190°C).
2. **Cook the Noodles:**

- If using regular lasagna noodles, cook them according to package instructions until al dente. Drain and set aside. If using no-boil noodles, skip this step.

3. **Prepare the Vegetable Filling:**
    - In a large skillet, heat olive oil over medium heat. Add the chopped onion and sauté until translucent (about 3-4 minutes).
    - Add the minced garlic and cook for an additional minute.
    - Stir in the diced zucchini, bell pepper, and mushrooms. Cook until the vegetables are tender (about 5-7 minutes).
    - Add the fresh spinach and cook until wilted. Season with oregano, basil, salt, and pepper. Remove from heat.

4. **Mix the Cheese Filling:**
    - In a bowl, combine ricotta cheese, Parmesan cheese, egg, and parsley (if using). Mix until well combined. Season with salt and pepper.

5. **Assemble the Lasagna:**
    - Spread a thin layer of marinara sauce on the bottom of a 9x13 inch baking dish.
    - Layer 3-4 lasagna noodles over the sauce.
    - Spread half of the ricotta mixture over the noodles, followed by half of the vegetable mixture, and a layer of marinara sauce.
    - Repeat the layers: noodles, remaining ricotta mixture, remaining vegetables, and more marinara sauce.
    - Top with a final layer of noodles and the remaining marinara sauce. Sprinkle with shredded mozzarella cheese.

6. **Bake:**
    - Cover the baking dish with foil (to prevent sticking, spray the foil with cooking spray) and bake for 25 minutes.
    - Remove the foil and bake for an additional 15-20 minutes, or until the cheese is bubbly and golden.

7. **Serve:**
    - Let the lasagna cool for about 10 minutes before slicing. Serve warm.

Cooking and Prep Time

- **Prep Time:** 20 minutes
- **Cook Time:** 45-50 minutes
- **Total Time:** 1 hour 10 minutes
- **Servings:** 6-8

Nutrition (per serving)

- **Calories:** Approximately 320
- **Total Fat:** 15g
- **Saturated Fat:** 7g
- **Cholesterol:** 70mg
- **Sodium:** 600mg
- **Total Carbohydrates:** 35g
- **Dietary Fiber:** 4g
- **Total Sugars:** 6g
- **Protein:** 18g

6.10 Herb-Crusted Tilapia

Ingredients

- 4 tilapia fillets
- 1 cup breadcrumbs (panko or regular)
- 2 tablespoons fresh parsley, chopped
- 1 tablespoon fresh dill, chopped (or 1 teaspoon dried dill)
- 1 tablespoon fresh basil, chopped (or 1 teaspoon dried basil)
- 2 cloves garlic, minced
- 1 lemon, zested and juiced
- 2 tablespoons olive oil
- Salt and pepper to taste
- Lemon wedges for serving

Directions

1. **Preheat the Oven**:
    - Preheat your oven to 400°F (200°C).
2. **Prepare the Herb Mixture**:
    - In a bowl, combine breadcrumbs, parsley, dill, basil, minced garlic, lemon zest, olive oil, salt, and pepper. Mix until well combined.
3. **Prepare the Tilapia**:
    - Place the tilapia fillets on a baking sheet lined with parchment paper. Drizzle with lemon juice and season with salt and pepper.
4. **Coat the Tilapia**:
    - Evenly distribute the herb and breadcrumb mixture over the top of each tilapia fillet, pressing down gently to adhere.
5. **Bake**:
    - Bake in the preheated oven for 12-15 minutes, or until the fish is cooked through and flakes easily with a fork.

6. **Serve**:
    - Remove from the oven and serve immediately with lemon wedges on the side.

Cooking and Prep Time

- **Prep Time:** 10 minutes
- **Cook Time:** 15 minutes
- **Total Time:** 25 minutes
- **Servings:** 4

Nutrition (per serving)

- **Calories:** Approximately 220
- **Total Fat:** 9g
- **Saturated Fat:** 1g
- **Cholesterol:** 70mg
- **Sodium:** 350mg
- **Total Carbohydrates:** 18g
- **Dietary Fiber:** 1g
- **Total Sugars:** 1g
- **Protein:** 22g

6.11 Balsamic Glazed Pork Chops

Ingredients

- 4 boneless pork chops (about 1 inch thick)
- 1 tablespoon olive oil
- Salt and pepper to taste
- 1/2 cup balsamic vinegar
- 2 tablespoons honey
- 2 cloves garlic, minced
- 1 teaspoon dried thyme (or 1 tablespoon fresh thyme)
- 1 teaspoon Dijon mustard
- Fresh parsley for garnish (optional)

Directions

1. **Prepare the Pork Chops**:
    - Pat the pork chops dry with paper towels. Season both sides with salt and pepper.
2. **Sear the Pork Chops**:
    - In a large skillet, heat olive oil over medium-high heat.
    - Add the pork chops and sear for about 4-5 minutes on each side until they are golden brown and cooked through (internal temperature should reach 145°F or 63°C). Remove the pork chops from the skillet and set aside.
3. **Make the Balsamic Glaze**:
    - In the same skillet, add the balsamic vinegar, honey, minced garlic, thyme, and Dijon mustard.
    - Bring the mixture to a simmer, scraping up any browned bits from the bottom of the skillet. Let it cook for about 5-7 minutes until the glaze thickens slightly.

4. **Glaze the Pork Chops**:
   - Return the pork chops to the skillet, spooning the balsamic glaze over them. Cook for an additional 1-2 minutes to heat through and coat the chops with the glaze.
5. **Serve**:
   - Remove from heat and garnish with fresh parsley if desired. Serve the pork chops with the balsamic glaze drizzled over the top.

Cooking and Prep Time

- **Prep Time:** 10 minutes
- **Cook Time:** 15 minutes
- **Total Time:** 25 minutes
- **Servings:** 4

Nutrition (per serving)

- **Calories:** Approximately 290
- **Total Fat:** 10g
- **Saturated Fat:** 2g
- **Cholesterol:** 90mg
- **Sodium:** 350mg
- **Total Carbohydrates:** 15g
- **Dietary Fiber:** 0g
- **Total Sugars:** 10g
- **Protein:** 30g

6.12 Stuffed Eggplant

Ingredients

- 2 large eggplants (about 350g each)
- 1 tablespoon olive oil
- 1 onion, chopped
- 2 garlic cloves, crushed
- 2 teaspoons Moroccan seasoning (or spices of your choice)
- 300g ground lamb or beef (or a vegetarian alternative)
- 1 can (400g) diced tomatoes
- 1/2 cup breadcrumbs
- 1/2 cup grated cheese (optional)
- Salt and pepper to taste

Directions

1. **Prepare the Eggplants**: Preheat the oven to 180°C (350°F). Cut the eggplants in half lengthwise and scoop out some of the flesh, leaving about a 1/4-inch rim. This can be chopped and added to the filling.
2. **Sweat the Eggplants**: Sprinkle the insides of the eggplant halves with salt and let them sit for about 30 minutes to draw out moisture. Rinse and pat dry.
3. **Cook the Filling**: In a skillet, heat the olive oil over medium heat. Add the chopped onion and crushed garlic, sautéing until softened. Add the ground meat and cook until browned. Stir in the chopped eggplant flesh, diced tomatoes, and Moroccan seasoning. Cook for an additional 5-10 minutes until the mixture is well combined. Season with salt and pepper.
4. **Assemble the Dish**: Spoon the filling into the eggplant halves. Top with breadcrumbs and cheese if using.
5. **Bake**: Place the stuffed eggplants on a baking sheet and bake in the preheated oven for about 30-35 minutes, or until the eggplants are tender and the tops are golden brown.

Cooking and Prep Time

- **Prep Time**: 15-20 minutes
- **Cooking Time**: 30-35 minutes
- **Total Time**: Approximately 1 hour

Serving Suggestions

This recipe serves 4 as a main dish. It pairs well with a side salad or some crusty bread.

For a more substantial meal, serve with couscous or rice.

Nutritional Information (per serving)

- Calories: Approximately 350-400 (depending on the meat and cheese used)
- Protein: 20-25g
- Carbohydrates: 30-35g
- Fat: 15-20g

6.13 Ratatouille

Ingredients

- **Vegetables:**
    - 2 medium eggplants, sliced
    - 2 zucchinis, sliced
    - 2 yellow squashes, sliced
    - 1 red bell pepper, diced
    - 1 yellow bell pepper, diced
    - 6 Roma tomatoes, sliced or 28 oz crushed tomatoes
- **Sauce:**
    - 4 tablespoons olive oil (divided)
    - 1 medium onion, diced
    - 4 cloves garlic, minced
    - 1/3 cup shredded carrot (optional)
    - 2 teaspoons dried basil
    - 1/2 teaspoon dried oregano
    - Salt and pepper to taste
- **Garnish:**
    - Fresh basil or parsley, chopped

Directions

1. **Preheat the Oven**: Preheat your oven to 375°F (190°C).
2. **Prepare the Sauce**: In a large skillet, heat 2 tablespoons of olive oil over medium heat. Add the diced onion, minced garlic, and shredded carrot (if using). Sauté until the vegetables are tender, about 5 minutes.
3. **Add Tomatoes**: Stir in the crushed tomatoes (or fresh sliced tomatoes) and season with salt, pepper, basil, and oregano. Let the sauce simmer for about 15 minutes until it thickens slightly.

4. **Layer the Vegetables**: In a baking dish, spread the tomato sauce evenly on the bottom. Arrange the sliced eggplant, zucchini, yellow squash, and bell peppers in an overlapping circular pattern over the sauce.
5. **Drizzle Olive Oil**: Brush the arranged vegetables with the remaining olive oil and sprinkle with salt and pepper.
6. **Bake**: Cover the dish with parchment paper and bake in the preheated oven for about 30 minutes. Then, remove the cover and bake for an additional 15-30 minutes, or until the vegetables are tender and the top is slightly caramelized.
7. **Serve**: Let the ratatouille cool for a few minutes before serving. Garnish with fresh basil or parsley. It can be served warm or at room temperature.

Cooking and Prep Time

- **Prep Time**: 30 minutes
- **Cook Time**: 1 hour
- **Total Time**: 1 hour 30 minutes

Serving Suggestions

This recipe serves approximately 6-8 people. Ratatouille can be enjoyed on its own, served with crusty bread, over pasta, or as a side dish to grilled meats or fish.

Nutritional Information (per serving)

- **Calories**: Approximately 106
- **Fat**: 3g
- **Carbohydrates**: 19g
- **Protein**: 3g
- **Fiber**: 4g

6.14 Moroccan Lentil Stew

Ingredients

- 2 tablespoons olive oil
- 1 onion, chopped
- 2 carrots, peeled and chopped
- 2 celery stalks, chopped
- 4 garlic cloves, minced
- 2 teaspoons ground cumin
- 1 teaspoon ground coriander
- 1 teaspoon paprika
- 1/2 teaspoon ground cinnamon
- 1/4 teaspoon red pepper flakes (optional)
- 1 cup green or brown lentils, rinsed
- 1 (28 oz) can crushed tomatoes
- 4 cups vegetable or chicken broth
- 1 bay leaf
- Salt and black pepper to taste
- 1/4 cup chopped fresh cilantro or parsley (for garnish)

Directions

1. In a large pot or Dutch oven, heat the olive oil over medium heat. Add the onion, carrots, and celery. Cook for about 5 minutes, stirring occasionally, until the vegetables start to soften.
2. Add the garlic, cumin, coriander, paprika, cinnamon, and red pepper flakes (if using). Cook for 1 minute, stirring constantly, until fragrant.
3. Stir in the lentils, crushed tomatoes, broth, and bay leaf. Season with salt and pepper to taste.
4. Bring the mixture to a boil, then reduce the heat to low. Simmer for 25-30 minutes, or until the lentils are tender and the stew has thickened.

5. Remove the bay leaf. Taste and adjust seasoning if necessary.
6. Serve the Moroccan lentil stew hot, garnished with chopped cilantro or parsley. It pairs well with crusty bread or couscous.

Cooking and Prep Time

- **Prep Time**: 15 minutes
- **Cook Time**: 35 minutes
- **Total Time**: 50 minutes

Serving Suggestions

This recipe serves 4-6 people as a main dish. It can also be served as a side dish or appetizer. For a heartier meal, consider adding diced cooked chicken or lamb.

Nutrition Information (per serving)

- **Calories**: 300
- **Fat**: 8g
- **Carbohydrates**: 45g
- **Protein**: 16g
- **Fiber**: 12g

Chapter 6: Snack and Appetizer Recipes

7.1 Hummus with Fresh Vegetables

Ingredients

- 1 (15 oz) can chickpeas, drained and rinsed
- 1/2 cup tahini
- 1/4 cup lemon juice (about 1 lemon)
- 2 cloves garlic
- 2 tbsp olive oil, plus more for drizzling
- 1/4 cup cold water
- 1 tsp salt
- 1/2 tsp cumin
- 2 tbsp diced cucumbers
- 2 tbsp diced yellow bell pepper
- 2 tbsp diced red bell pepper
- 2 tbsp diced grape tomatoes
- Chopped parsley for garnish
- Pita chips, crackers, and cut up vegetables for serving

Instructions

1. In a food processor, combine the chickpeas, tahini, lemon juice, garlic, olive oil, water, salt, and cumin. Blend until smooth and creamy, about 2-3 minutes, scraping down the sides as needed.
2. Taste and adjust seasoning if desired, adding more lemon juice for brightness or salt to taste.
3. Transfer the hummus to a shallow bowl or plate. Use the back of a spoon to create a well in the center.
4. Top with the diced cucumbers, bell peppers, and tomatoes. Drizzle with olive oil and sprinkle with chopped parsley.

5. Serve immediately with pita chips, crackers, and cut up vegetables for dipping.

Prep Time: 10 minutes

Total Time: 10 minutes

Servings: 6-8

Nutrition (per serving)

- Calories: 123
- Carbs: 3g
- Protein: 3g
- Fat: 12g
- Fiber: 2g

7.2 Greek Yogurt with Berries

Ingredients

- 1 cup plain Greek yogurt
- 1/2 cup mixed berries (such as strawberries, blueberries, and raspberries)
- 1 tablespoon honey (optional)
- 1 tablespoon chopped nuts (such as walnuts or almonds, optional)
- Fresh mint leaves for garnish (optional)

Directions

1. **Prepare the Berries**: Wash the berries thoroughly. If using strawberries, remove the stems and slice them into halves or quarters.
2. **Assemble the Dish**: In a bowl, add the Greek yogurt. Top it with the mixed berries.
3. **Add Sweetness**: Drizzle honey over the top if desired.
4. **Add Crunch**: Sprinkle chopped nuts on top for added texture and flavor.
5. **Garnish**: Add fresh mint leaves for a refreshing touch, if using.
6. **Serve**: Enjoy immediately as a nutritious breakfast or snack.

Prep Time

- **Prep Time**: 5 minutes
- **Total Time**: 5 minutes

Serving Suggestions

This recipe serves 1 person but can easily be multiplied for more servings. It pairs well with granola or can be enjoyed as a parfait layered in a glass.

Nutritional Information (per serving)

- **Calories**: Approximately 220-250 kcal (depending on honey and nuts used)
- **Total Fat**: 4-9g (varies with nuts)
- **Saturated Fat**: 1g
- **Carbohydrates**: 35-45g

- **Protein**: 14-19g
- **Dietary Fiber**: 2-4g
- **Sugars**: 20-30g (includes natural sugars from fruit and honey)

7.3 Roasted Chickpeas

Ingredients

- 2 (15-ounce) cans chickpeas, drained and rinsed
- 2 tablespoons olive oil
- 1 teaspoon garlic powder
- 1 teaspoon paprika
- 1/2 teaspoon cumin
- 1/4 teaspoon cayenne pepper (optional)
- 1/2 teaspoon salt

Directions

1. **Preheat the oven** to 400°F (200°C). Line a baking sheet with parchment paper.
2. **Pat the chickpeas dry** with paper towels or a clean kitchen towel. Remove any loose skins.
3. **In a large bowl**, toss the chickpeas with olive oil, garlic powder, paprika, cumin, cayenne (if using), and salt until evenly coated.
4. **Spread the chickpeas** in a single layer on the prepared baking sheet.
5. **Roast for 20-25 minutes**, stirring halfway, until golden brown and crispy.
6. **Remove from the oven** and let cool completely on the baking sheet. The chickpeas will continue to crisp up as they cool.
7. **Once cooled**, transfer to an airtight container and store at room temperature for up to 1 week.

Cooking and Prep Time

- **Prep Time**: 5 minutes
- **Cook Time**: 20-25 minutes
- **Total Time**: 25-30 minutes

Serving Suggestions

- Enjoy the roasted chickpeas as a snack by the handful

- Add to salads, grain bowls, or soups for extra crunch and protein
- Use as a topping for avocado toast or hummus

Nutrition Information (per 1/2 cup serving)

- **Calories**: 150
- **Fat**: 5g
- **Carbohydrates**: 20g
- **Protein**: 6g
- **Fiber**: 5g

7.4 Avocado Toast

Ingredients

- 1 ripe avocado
- 2 slices of bread (sourdough, whole grain, or your choice)
- 1/2 lemon (for juice)
- Salt and pepper to taste
- Optional toppings:
    - Red pepper flakes
    - Olive oil
    - Fresh herbs (like cilantro or parsley)
    - Sliced tomatoes
    - Poached or fried egg
    - Feta cheese

Directions

1. **Toast the Bread**: Begin by toasting your slices of bread to your desired level of crispiness.
2. **Prepare the Avocado**: While the bread is toasting, cut the avocado in half and remove the pit. Scoop the flesh into a bowl.
3. **Mash the Avocado**: Add the juice of half a lemon, salt, and pepper to the avocado. Mash it with a fork to your desired consistency (smooth or chunky).
4. **Assemble the Toast**: Once the bread is toasted, spread the mashed avocado generously on each slice.
5. **Add Toppings**: Drizzle with olive oil if desired, and add any additional toppings you like, such as red pepper flakes, herbs, sliced tomatoes, or a poached egg.
6. **Serve**: Enjoy immediately while the toast is still warm.

Cooking and Prep Time

- **Prep Time**: 5 minutes
- **Cook Time**: 5 minutes
- **Total Time**: 10 minutes

Serving Suggestions

This recipe serves 1-2 people, depending on appetite. Avocado toast can be enjoyed on its own or paired with a smoothie or salad for a more filling meal.

Nutritional Information (per serving)

- **Calories**: Approximately 250-300 kcal (depending on bread and toppings)
- **Total Fat**: 15g
- **Carbohydrates**: 30g
- **Protein**: 6g
- **Fiber**: 7g

7.5 Apple Slices with Peanut Butter

Ingredients

- 2 medium apples (any variety, such as Gala or Red Delicious), cored and sliced
- 2 tablespoons peanut butter (creamy or chunky)
- Optional toppings:
    - 1 handful of raspberries, halved
    - 2 bananas, thinly sliced
    - 2 tablespoons runny honey
    - 2 tablespoons mixed nuts, seeds, or raisins

Directions

1. **Prepare the Apples**: Wash the apples thoroughly. Core and slice them into ¼-inch thick slices.
2. **Spread Peanut Butter**: Place the apple slices on a plate or platter. Spread a tablespoon of peanut butter on one side of each apple slice.
3. **Add Toppings**: If desired, arrange the optional toppings (raspberries, banana slices, nuts, etc.) on top of the peanut butter.
4. **Drizzle with Honey**: For added sweetness, drizzle honey over the topped apple slices.
5. **Serve**: Enjoy immediately as a healthy snack!

Prep Time

- **Prep Time**: 5 minutes
- **Total Time**: 5 minutes

Serving Suggestions

This recipe serves about 2-4 people, depending on the number of apple slices and appetites. It can be served as a snack, breakfast, or even a light dessert.

Nutritional Information (per serving)

- **Calories**: Approximately 209 kcal
- **Total Fat**: 7g
- **Carbohydrates**: 38g
- **Protein**: 4g
- **Fiber**: 5g
- **Sugar**: 26g
- **Sodium**: 39mg
- **Potassium**: 390mg

7.6 Cucumber Sandwiches

Ingredients

- 1 English cucumber, thinly sliced
- 8 slices soft white bread (such as Pepperidge Farm)
- 4 ounces cream cheese, softened
- 2 tablespoons mayonnaise
- 1 tablespoon finely chopped fresh dill (or 1 teaspoon dried dill)
- 1/4 teaspoon salt
- 1/8 teaspoon black pepper

Directions

1. **In a small bowl**, mix together the cream cheese, mayonnaise, dill, salt, and pepper until well combined.
2. **Spread the cream cheese mixture** evenly on one side of each slice of bread.
3. **Layer the cucumber slices** on top of the cream cheese on 4 of the bread slices.
4. **Top with the remaining 4 bread slices**, cream cheese side down, to make 4 sandwiches.
5. **Using a serrated knife**, gently cut off the crusts from each sandwich.
6. **Cut each sandwich** into quarters or halves, depending on your desired size.
7. **Arrange the cucumber sandwiches** on a serving platter and serve chilled or at room temperature.

Cooking and Prep Time

- **Prep Time**: 15 minutes
- **Total Time**: 15 minutes

Serving Suggestions

This recipe makes 16 quarter sandwiches or 8 half sandwiches, serving 4-8 people as an appetizer. Cucumber sandwiches are perfect for tea parties, bridal showers, or as a light snack.

Nutrition Information (per serving)

- **Calories**: 100
- **Fat**: 5g
- **Carbohydrates**: 12g
- **Protein**: 2g
- **Sodium**: 200mg
- **Fiber**: 1g

7.7 Edamame

Ingredients

- 2 cups edamame (in pods, fresh or frozen)
- 1 teaspoon sea salt (plus more for serving)
- Optional toppings:
    - Red pepper flakes
    - Sesame oil
    - Soy sauce
    - Lemon or lime juice

Directions

1. **Boil Water**: In a large pot, bring water to a boil. Add a teaspoon of sea salt to the water.
2. **Cook Edamame**: Add the edamame pods to the boiling water. If using frozen edamame, cook for about 5 minutes; if fresh, cook for about 3-4 minutes. The edamame should be tender but still firm.
3. **Drain and Rinse**: Drain the edamame in a colander and rinse under cold water to stop the cooking process.
4. **Season**: Transfer the edamame to a serving bowl. Sprinkle with additional sea salt and any optional toppings you prefer, such as red pepper flakes or a drizzle of sesame oil.
5. **Serve**: Serve warm or at room temperature. To eat, simply squeeze the pods to pop the beans into your mouth.

Cooking and Prep Time

- **Prep Time**: 5 minutes
- **Cook Time**: 5 minutes
- **Total Time**: 10 minutes

Serving Suggestions

This recipe serves 2-4 people as a snack or appetizer. Edamame can be enjoyed on their own or served alongside sushi, salads, or grain bowls.

Nutritional Information (per serving, 1 cup cooked)

- **Calories**: Approximately 190
- **Total Fat**: 8g
- **Saturated Fat**: 1g
- **Carbohydrates**: 14g
- **Protein**: 17g
- **Fiber**: 8g
- **Sodium**: 300mg (if salted)

7.8 Rice Cakes with Almond Butter

Ingredients

- 2 plain rice cakes
- 2 tablespoons almond butter
- 1 banana, sliced (optional)
- 1 tablespoon honey or maple syrup (optional)
- A sprinkle of cinnamon (optional)
- Chopped nuts or seeds for topping (optional)

Directions

1. **Spread Almond Butter**: Take the rice cakes and spread 1 tablespoon of almond butter on each cake, ensuring an even layer.
2. **Add Banana Slices**: If using, arrange the banana slices on top of the almond butter for added sweetness and nutrition.
3. **Drizzle Sweetener**: If desired, drizzle honey or maple syrup over the banana slices for extra flavor.
4. **Sprinkle Cinnamon**: Add a sprinkle of cinnamon for a warm, aromatic touch.
5. **Top with Nuts/Seeds**: For added crunch and nutrition, sprinkle chopped nuts or seeds on top.
6. **Serve**: Enjoy immediately as a healthy snack or breakfast!

Cooking and Prep Time

- **Prep Time**: 5 minutes
- **Total Time**: 5 minutes

Serving Suggestions

This recipe serves 1-2 people, depending on how many rice cakes are prepared. It can be enjoyed as a snack, breakfast, or a light dessert.

Nutritional Information (per serving, 2 rice cakes with almond butter)

- **Calories**: Approximately 300-350 kcal (depending on toppings)

- **Total Fat**: 18g
- **Saturated Fat**: 1.5g
- **Carbohydrates**: 30g
- **Protein**: 8g
- **Fiber**: 4g
- **Sugar**: 5-10g (includes natural sugars from banana and honey)

7.9 Vegetable Spring Rolls

Ingredients

- **For the Filling:**
    - 3 cups shredded cabbage
    - 1 medium carrot, shredded
    - 1/4 cup bell pepper (red or green), julienned
    - 1/2 cup bean sprouts (optional)
    - 2 green onions, chopped (white and green parts separated)
    - 1-2 teaspoons oil (for sautéing)
    - 1-2 teaspoons soy sauce
    - 1 teaspoon rice vinegar
    - 1/4 teaspoon black pepper
    - Salt to taste (if needed)
- **For the Spring Rolls:**
    - 6-10 spring roll wrappers (available in Asian grocery stores)
    - Oil for deep frying or a small amount for baking

Directions

1. **Prepare the Filling**:
    - Heat oil in a large pan or wok over medium-high heat.
    - Add the white parts of the green onions and sauté for about 1 minute.
    - Add the shredded cabbage, carrots, bell pepper, and bean sprouts. Stir-fry until the vegetables are tender but still crunchy, about 3-4 minutes.
    - Stir in the soy sauce, rice vinegar, black pepper, and salt. Remove from heat and let the mixture cool.
2. **Assemble the Spring Rolls**:
    - Lay a spring roll wrapper on a clean surface with one corner pointing towards you (like a diamond shape).

- Place about 2 tablespoons of the vegetable filling near the bottom corner of the wrapper.
- Fold the bottom corner over the filling, then fold in the sides, and roll tightly towards the top corner. Use a little water to seal the edge.

3. **Cook the Spring Rolls**:
   - **For Frying**: Heat oil in a deep pan until hot. Carefully add the spring rolls (in batches) and fry for about 2-3 minutes or until golden brown. Remove and drain on paper towels.
   - **For Baking**: Preheat the oven to 400°F (200°C). Place the spring rolls on a baking sheet and lightly brush with oil. Bake for about 20-25 minutes, turning halfway through, until golden and crispy.
4. **Serve**:
   - Serve the spring rolls hot with dipping sauces like sweet chili sauce, soy sauce, or hoisin sauce.

Cooking and Prep Time

- **Prep Time**: 15 minutes
- **Cook Time**: 10-25 minutes (depending on frying or baking)
- **Total Time**: 25-40 minutes

Serving Suggestions

This recipe makes about 6-10 spring rolls, serving 2-4 people as an appetizer or snack. Pair with a salad or soup for a light meal.

Nutritional Information (per spring roll, fried)

- **Calories**: Approximately 150-170 kcal
- **Total Fat**: 8g
- **Saturated Fat**: 1g
- **Carbohydrates**: 18g
- **Protein**: 3g
- **Fiber**: 2g

- **Sodium**: 200mg

7.10 Cheese and Crackers

Ingredients

- 6 ounces sharp cheddar cheese, shredded (about 1.5 cups)
- 1 cup all-purpose flour (125g)
- 1.5 teaspoons cornstarch
- 1/4 teaspoon salt
- 6 tablespoons unsalted butter, cold and cut into pieces (85g)
- 2 tablespoons cold water (optional)
- Sea salt for sprinkling on top (optional)

Directions

1. In a food processor, combine the shredded cheddar cheese, flour, cornstarch, and salt. Pulse until mixed (about 30 seconds).
2. Add the cold butter and pulse until the mixture resembles wet sand (about 20 seconds).
3. If the dough is too dry, add cold water gradually until large clumps form (about 10 pulses).
4. Transfer the dough to a lightly floured surface, divide it in half, and pat each half into a square about 6 inches wide.
5. Wrap each square in plastic wrap and refrigerate for at least 45 minutes (up to 2 days).
6. Preheat the oven to 350°F (177°C) and line two large baking sheets with parchment paper.
7. Unwrap the dough and roll each square into a larger square (about 9 inches).
8. Trim the edges to form a neat square, then cut into 1-inch squares or rectangles.
9. Place the cut squares on the prepared baking sheets. Use a skewer to poke a hole in the center of each cracker and sprinkle with sea salt if desired.
10. Bake for 16-20 minutes, rotating the sheets halfway through, until golden brown. For crunchier crackers, bake for an additional 2-4 minutes.

11. Allow the crackers to cool completely on the baking sheets before serving. Store in an airtight container at room temperature for up to one week.

Cooking and Prep Time

- Prep Time: 15 minutes (excluding chilling time)
- Cooking Time: 16-20 minutes
- Chilling Time: 45 minutes

Serving Suggestions

These cheese crackers can be enjoyed on their own or served with dips, soups, or alongside a cheese platter. They are perfect for parties, school lunches, or as a quick snack.

Nutritional Information (per serving, based on 64 crackers)

- Calories: Approximately 50
- Protein: 1.5g
- Carbohydrates: 5g
- Fat: 3g
- Sodium: 50mg

7.11 Popcorn with Nutritional Yeast

Ingredients

- 1/2 cup unpopped popcorn kernels
- 2 tablespoons coconut oil or vegetable oil
- 1/4 cup nutritional yeast
- 1/2 teaspoon salt (or to taste)

Directions

1. In a large pot or dutch oven, heat 1 tablespoon of the oil over medium-high heat.
2. Add the popcorn kernels in a single layer and cover with a lid.
3. Cook, shaking the pot occasionally, until the popping slows to 2-3 seconds between pops (about 2-3 minutes).
4. Remove from heat and transfer the popped popcorn to a large bowl.
5. Add the remaining 1 tablespoon oil, nutritional yeast, and salt. Toss to coat evenly.
6. Serve immediately while warm.

Cooking and Prep Time

- Prep Time: 5 minutes
- Cooking Time: 2-3 minutes

Serving Suggestions

This popcorn makes a great snack on its own or can be served alongside your favorite movie or TV show. The nutritional yeast adds a savory, "cheesy" flavor that is sure to satisfy your cravings.

Nutrition Information (per serving, based on 4 servings)

- Calories: 150
- Total Fat: 9g
- Saturated Fat: 7g
- Sodium: 300mg

- Total Carbohydrates: 15g
- Dietary Fiber: 3g
- Protein: 5g

7.12 Fruit Salad

Ingredients

For the Dressing

- 1/4 cup honey
- 1/4 cup freshly squeezed orange juice
- Zest of 1 lemon

For the Salad

- 1 lb strawberries, hulled and quartered
- 6 oz blueberries
- 6 oz raspberries
- 3 kiwis, peeled and sliced
- 1 orange, peeled and cut into wedges
- 2 apples, peeled and chopped
- 1 mango, peeled and chopped
- 2 cups grapes, halved

Directions

1. **Make the Dressing**: In a small bowl, whisk together the honey, orange juice, and lemon zest until well combined.
2. **Prepare the Fruit**: In a large bowl, add the strawberries, blueberries, raspberries, kiwis, orange wedges, apples, mango, and grapes.
3. **Combine**: Pour the dressing over the fruit and gently toss to combine, ensuring all the fruit is coated.
4. **Chill**: Refrigerate the fruit salad for about 30 minutes before serving to allow the flavors to meld.

Prep Time

- **Prep Time**: 15 minutes
- **Total Time**: 20 minutes (including chilling)

Serving Suggestions

This fruit salad can be served as a side dish, a light dessert, or a healthy snack. It's perfect for summer gatherings, picnics, or as a refreshing treat any time of year.

Nutritional Information (per serving, based on 8 servings)

- **Calories**: Approximately 178
- **Total Fat**: 0.5g
- **Saturated Fat**: 0g
- **Sodium**: 5mg
- **Total Carbohydrates**: 45g
- **Dietary Fiber**: 5g
- **Sugars**: 30g
- **Protein**: 1g

7.13 Kale Chips

Ingredients

- 1 large bundle of kale (curly or lacinato)
- 1-2 tablespoons melted coconut oil or olive oil
- Seasonings of choice (e.g., sea salt, garlic powder, nutritional yeast, chili powder, or parmesan cheese)

Directions

1. **Preheat the Oven**: Preheat your oven to 300°F (150°C).
2. **Prepare the Kale**: Rinse the kale thoroughly and dry it completely. Remove the tough stems and tear the leaves into bite-sized pieces.
3. **Season the Kale**: In a large mixing bowl, drizzle the kale with melted oil and sprinkle your chosen seasonings. Toss the kale gently with your hands to ensure even coating.
4. **Arrange on Baking Sheet**: Spread the seasoned kale in a single layer on a baking sheet, ensuring that the pieces do not overlap to promote even crisping.
5. **Bake**: Bake in the preheated oven for about 10 minutes. After 10 minutes, rotate the baking sheet and bake for an additional 10-15 minutes, or until the kale is crispy and slightly golden. Keep a close eye to prevent burning.
6. **Cool and Serve**: Remove the kale chips from the oven and let them cool for a few minutes. They will become crispier as they cool. Enjoy immediately or store in an airtight container.

Prep Time

- **Prep Time**: 10 minutes
- **Cooking Time**: 20-25 minutes

Serving Suggestions

Kale chips can be enjoyed as a standalone snack, or served as a crunchy topping for salads and soups. They are perfect for parties or as a healthy snack option for kids.

Nutritional Information (per serving, based on 4 servings)

- **Calories**: Approximately 61
- **Total Fat**: 4g
- **Saturated Fat**: 1g
- **Sodium**: 83mg
- **Total Carbohydrates**: 4g
- **Dietary Fiber**: 2g
- **Sugars**: 0g
- **Protein**: 3g
- **Vitamin A**: 4360 IU
- **Vitamin C**: 52.8 mg
- **Calcium**: 119 mg
- **Iron**: 0.7 mg

7.14 Deviled Eggs

Ingredients

- 6 large eggs
- 1/4 cup mayonnaise
- 1 tablespoon Dijon mustard (or yellow mustard)
- 1 tablespoon sweet pickle relish (or diced dill pickle)
- Salt and pepper, to taste
- Paprika for garnish

Directions

1. **Hard Boil the Eggs**: Place the eggs in a saucepan and cover them with cold water, ensuring there's about 1.5 inches of water above the eggs. Bring the water to a boil over medium-high heat. Once boiling, cover the pot, remove it from heat, and let it sit for 12-14 minutes.
2. **Cool the Eggs**: After the time is up, transfer the eggs to an ice water bath to cool for about 5-10 minutes. This will make peeling easier.
3. **Peel and Slice**: Once cooled, gently tap the eggs on a hard surface to crack the shell, then peel them under running water if needed. Slice each egg in half lengthwise and carefully remove the yolks, placing them in a mixing bowl.
4. **Make the Filling**: Mash the yolks with a fork until smooth. Add mayonnaise, mustard, pickle relish, salt, and pepper. Mix until well combined and creamy. Adjust seasoning to taste.
5. **Fill the Egg Whites**: Spoon or pipe the yolk mixture back into the hollowed egg whites.
6. **Garnish and Serve**: Sprinkle paprika on top for garnish. Serve immediately or refrigerate until ready to serve.

Cooking and Prep Time

- **Prep Time**: 15 minutes

- **Cooking Time**: 12-14 minutes (plus cooling time)

Serving Suggestions

Deviled eggs can be served as an appetizer at parties, picnics, or holiday gatherings. They pair well with other finger foods and can be made in advance for convenience.

Nutritional Information (per serving, based on 6 servings)

- **Calories**: Approximately 70
- **Total Fat**: 5g
- **Saturated Fat**: 1g
- **Cholesterol**: 186mg
- **Sodium**: 60mg
- **Total Carbohydrates**: 1g
- **Dietary Fiber**: 0g
- **Sugars**: 0g
- **Protein**: 6g

Chapter 7: Dessert Recipes

8.1 Berry Parfait

Ingredients (for 2 servings)

- 1 cup Greek yogurt (280 g)
- ½ cup granola (120 g)
- 1 banana, sliced
- ½ cup strawberries, hulled and quartered (75 g)
- ½ cup raspberries (60 g)
- ½ cup blueberries (50 g)
- Honey (to taste)

Directions

1. **Prepare the Ingredients**: Wash and prepare all the fruits by hulling the strawberries and slicing the banana.
2. **Layer the Parfait**:
    - In two glasses, start by adding half of the Greek yogurt to each glass.
    - Add a layer of sliced bananas and strawberries on top of the yogurt.
    - Follow with another layer of yogurt, then sprinkle granola over it.
    - Add a layer of raspberries and blueberries.
3. **Finish**: Drizzle honey on top of the parfaits for added sweetness.
4. **Serve**: Enjoy immediately or refrigerate for a short time before serving.

Cooking and Prep Time

- **Prep Time**: 10 minutes
- **Cooking Time**: None (no cooking required)

Nutrition Information (per serving)

- **Calories**: 382

- **Fat**: 7 g
- **Carbohydrates**: 63 g
- **Fiber**: 8 g
- **Sugar**: 39 g
- **Protein**: 17 g

8.2 Rice Pudding

Ingredients (for 4 servings)

- 1 ½ cups cooked white rice (or ¾ cup uncooked rice)
- 2 cups whole milk (divided)
- ⅓ cup sugar
- ¼ teaspoon salt
- 1 large egg, beaten
- ½ teaspoon vanilla extract
- 1 tablespoon unsalted butter
- ½ teaspoon ground cinnamon (optional)
- ⅛ teaspoon ground nutmeg (optional)
- ⅔ cup golden raisins (optional)

Directions

1. **Cook the Rice**: If using uncooked rice, combine ¾ cup of rice with 1 ½ cups of cold water in a medium saucepan. Bring to a boil, then reduce the heat to low, cover, and simmer for about 18 minutes or until the water is absorbed. If using cooked rice, skip this step.
2. **Combine Ingredients**: In a nonstick saucepan, combine the cooked rice, 1 ½ cups of milk, sugar, and salt. Bring to a low boil over medium heat, stirring frequently.
3. **Thicken the Mixture**: Cook uncovered for about 15-20 minutes, stirring often until the mixture thickens and becomes creamy.
4. **Temper the Egg**: In a bowl, whisk the beaten egg with the remaining ½ cup of milk. Gradually add about 1 cup of the hot rice mixture to the egg while stirring to prevent the egg from scrambling.
5. **Finish Cooking**: Pour the egg mixture back into the saucepan with the remaining rice mixture. Stir in the raisins (if using) and cook for an additional 2 minutes.

6. **Add Flavor**: Remove from heat and stir in the butter, vanilla extract, and spices (cinnamon and nutmeg, if desired).
7. **Serve**: Serve warm, garnished with a sprinkle of cinnamon or nutmeg if desired.

Cooking and Prep Time

- **Prep Time**: 10 minutes
- **Cooking Time**: 30 minutes
- **Total Time**: 40 minutes

Nutrition Information (per serving)

- **Calories**: 210
- **Fat**: 5 g
- **Carbohydrates**: 36 g
- **Fiber**: 1 g
- **Sugar**: 10 g
- **Protein**: 6 g

8.3 Low-Sugar Apple Crisp

Ingredients (for 4 servings)

- **3 medium apples** (such as Granny Smith or Empire), cored and sliced
- **1 tablespoon sugar** (or a sugar substitute)
- **1 teaspoon ground cinnamon** (divided)
- **½ teaspoon lemon juice**
- **⅓ cup light brown sugar** (unpacked)
- **½ cup rolled oats** (gluten-free if needed)
- **½ cup almond flour**
- **¼ cup unsalted butter**, cut into small squares
- **Pinch of salt**

Directions

1. **Preheat the Oven**: Preheat your oven to 375°F (190°C).
2. **Prepare the Apples**: In a large bowl, combine the sliced apples with the sugar, ½ teaspoon of cinnamon, and lemon juice. Toss to coat the apples evenly and set aside.
3. **Grease the Baking Dish**: Lightly grease a standard loaf pan or an 8x8 inch baking dish.
4. **Assemble the Apple Layer**: Pour the apple mixture into the prepared baking dish, spreading it evenly.
5. **Make the Crisp Topping**: In a separate bowl, combine the remaining ½ teaspoon of cinnamon, light brown sugar, rolled oats, almond flour, butter, and a pinch of salt. Use your hands to mix until the mixture resembles wet sand.
6. **Top the Apples**: Sprinkle the crisp topping evenly over the apple layer.
7. **Bake**: Place the dish in the oven and bake for about 40-45 minutes, or until the topping is golden brown and the apples are bubbling.
8. **Cool and Serve**: Allow to cool for a few minutes before serving. Enjoy it warm, optionally with low-sugar ice cream or yogurt.

Cooking and Prep Time

- **Prep Time**: 15 minutes
- **Cooking Time**: 40-45 minutes
- **Total Time**: Approximately 60 minutes

Nutrition Information (per serving)

- **Calories**: 210
- **Fat**: 10 g
- **Carbohydrates**: 30 g
- **Fiber**: 3 g
- **Sugar**: 8 g (includes natural sugars from apples)
- **Protein**: 3 g

8.4 Coconut Macaroons

Ingredients (for 12-15 macaroons)

- 4 cups sweetened shredded coconut
- ⅞ cup sweetened condensed milk (approximately ¾ cup plus 2 tablespoons)
- 1 teaspoon vanilla extract
- 2 large egg whites
- ¼ teaspoon salt
- 4 ounces semi-sweet chocolate (optional, for dipping)

Directions

1. **Preheat the Oven**: Preheat your oven to 325°F (165°C). Line two baking sheets with parchment paper.
2. **Mix Coconut Ingredients**: In a medium bowl, combine the shredded coconut, sweetened condensed milk, and vanilla extract. Mix until well combined.
3. **Beat Egg Whites**: In a separate bowl, use an electric mixer to beat the egg whites and salt until stiff peaks form.
4. **Combine Mixtures**: Gently fold the beaten egg whites into the coconut mixture until fully incorporated.
5. **Shape the Macaroons**: Using a mini ice cream scoop or two spoons, form heaping tablespoons of the mixture into mounds on the prepared baking sheets, spacing them about 1 inch apart.
6. **Bake**: Bake for about 23-25 minutes, or until the tops and edges are golden brown. Rotate the pans halfway through baking for even cooking.
7. **Cool**: Allow the macaroons to cool on the baking sheets for a few minutes before transferring them to a wire rack to cool completely.
8. **Optional Chocolate Dip**: If desired, melt the chocolate in a microwave-safe bowl, stirring every 30 seconds until smooth. Dip the bottoms of the cooled macaroons in the chocolate and return them to the baking sheets. Refrigerate for about 10 minutes to set the chocolate.

Cooking and Prep Time

- **Prep Time**: 15 minutes
- **Cooking Time**: 25 minutes
- **Total Time**: Approximately 40 minutes

Nutrition Information (per macaroon, without chocolate)

- **Calories**: 120
- **Fat**: 5 g
- **Carbohydrates**: 18 g
- **Fiber**: 1 g
- **Sugar**: 10 g
- **Protein**: 2 g

8.5 Chia Seed Pudding

Ingredients (for 2 servings)

- **1 cup unsweetened almond milk** (or milk of your choice)
- **4 tablespoons chia seeds**
- **1 tablespoon maple syrup** (or honey, to taste)
- **½ teaspoon vanilla extract** (optional)
- **Pinch of cinnamon** (optional)

Directions

1. **In a bowl or jar with a lid**, combine the almond milk, chia seeds, maple syrup, vanilla extract (if using), and cinnamon (if using). Stir well to combine.
2. **Cover and refrigerate for at least 2 hours**, or up to 5 days. Stir the pudding occasionally to prevent clumping.
3. **When ready to serve**, stir the pudding again. It should have a thick, pudding-like consistency.
4. **Top with your favorite toppings**, such as fresh fruit, nuts, coconut flakes, or a drizzle of nut butter.

Cooking and Prep Time

- **Prep Time**: 5 minutes
- **Chilling Time**: 2 hours (minimum)
- **Total Time**: 2 hours 5 minutes

Nutrition Information (per serving)

- **Calories**: 150
- **Fat**: 7 g
- **Carbohydrates**: 19 g
- **Fiber**: 9 g
- **Sugar**: 7 g
- **Protein**: 5 g

8.6 Lemon Sorbet

Ingredients (for 4 servings)

- **1 ½ cups freshly squeezed lemon juice** (about 6-8 lemons)
- **1 ¼ cups water**
- **1 cup granulated sugar** (or a sugar substitute like erythritol)
- **1 tablespoon lemon zest**
- **Optional**: 1-2 tablespoons vodka (to improve texture)

Directions

1. **Make Simple Syrup**: In a saucepan, combine the water and sugar. Heat over medium heat, stirring until the sugar dissolves completely. Bring to a boil, then remove from heat and let cool.
2. **Add Lemon Ingredients**: Once the syrup has cooled, stir in the lemon juice and lemon zest. If using vodka, add it now. This helps the sorbet maintain a smoother texture.
3. **Chill the Mixture**: Refrigerate the lemon mixture for at least 2 hours until it's thoroughly chilled.
4. **Churn the Sorbet**: Pour the chilled mixture into an ice cream maker and churn according to the manufacturer's instructions, usually about 20-30 minutes, until it reaches a soft-serve consistency.
5. **Freeze**: Transfer the sorbet to a freezer-safe container and freeze for at least 3 hours to firm up.
6. **Serve**: Scoop the sorbet into bowls or hollowed-out lemon halves for a decorative touch. Garnish with fresh mint or lemon zest if desired.

Cooking and Prep Time

- **Prep Time**: 15 minutes
- **Chilling Time**: 2 hours
- **Churning and Freezing Time**: 3-4 hours

- **Total Time**: Approximately 5-6 hours

Nutrition Information (per serving)

- **Calories**: 120
- **Fat**: 0 g
- **Carbohydrates**: 31 g
- **Fiber**: 1 g
- **Sugar**: 28 g
- **Protein**: 0 g

8.7 Banana Ice Cream

Ingredients (for 4 servings)

- **4 ripe bananas**
- **½ cup milk** (dairy or non-dairy, such as almond or coconut milk)
- **½ cup heavy cream** (optional for creaminess)
- **2 tablespoons honey or maple syrup** (optional, adjust to taste)
- **1 teaspoon vanilla extract** (optional)

Directions

1. **Prepare the Bananas**: Peel the bananas and slice them into 1-inch pieces. Place the banana slices in a single layer on a baking sheet and freeze for at least 2 hours, or until solid.
2. **Blend the Ingredients**: Once the bananas are frozen, transfer them to a blender or food processor. Add the milk, heavy cream (if using), honey or maple syrup, and vanilla extract. Blend until smooth and creamy. You may need to stop and scrape down the sides a few times.
3. **Adjust Consistency**: If the mixture is too thick, add a little more milk until you reach your desired consistency.
4. **Serve Immediately or Freeze**: For a soft-serve consistency, serve the banana ice cream immediately. For a firmer texture, transfer it to an airtight container and freeze for an additional 1-2 hours.
5. **Enjoy**: Scoop into bowls and enjoy as is, or top with your favorite toppings like nuts, chocolate chips, or fresh fruit.

Cooking and Prep Time

- **Prep Time**: 10 minutes
- **Freezing Time**: 2 hours
- **Total Time**: Approximately 2 hours 10 minutes

Nutrition Information (per serving)

- **Calories**: 120
- **Fat**: 4 g (with heavy cream)
- **Carbohydrates**: 22 g
- **Fiber**: 2 g
- **Sugar**: 10 g (natural sugars from bananas)
- **Protein**: 2 g

8.8 Chocolate Avocado Mousse

Ingredients (for 2 servings)

- 1 medium ripe Haas avocado (about 4.5 ounces, peeled and pitted)
- ⅓ cup unsweetened cocoa powder (Dutch-processed for best flavor)
- ⅓ cup water (or milk of choice)
- 1 teaspoon pure vanilla extract
- 1 ½ teaspoons sweetener (such as stevia or maple syrup, adjust to taste)
- A pinch of salt

Directions

1. **Prepare the Ingredients**: In a food processor, combine the avocado, cocoa powder, water (or milk), vanilla extract, sweetener, and salt.
2. **Blend**: Process the mixture until smooth and creamy, about 1 minute. Stop to scrape down the sides of the bowl as needed to ensure everything is well combined.
3. **Taste and Adjust**: After blending, taste the mousse and adjust the sweetness or cocoa powder as desired.
4. **Rest**: Allow the mousse to rest at room temperature for about 30 minutes. This helps the flavors meld and improves the texture.
5. **Serve**: Spoon the mousse into serving dishes. You can enjoy it immediately or refrigerate it for a few hours before serving.

Cooking and Prep Time

- **Prep Time**: 10 minutes
- **Rest Time**: 30 minutes
- **Total Time**: 40 minutes

Nutrition Information (per serving)

- **Calories**: 149
- **Fat**: 9 g

- **Carbohydrates**: 18 g
- **Fiber**: 7 g
- **Sugar**: 2 g (natural sugars from avocado and sweetener)
- **Protein**: 2 g

8.9 Peach Cobbler

Ingredients (for 6 servings)

- 2 cups fresh peaches (peeled and sliced, or 1 (29-ounce) can of peaches, drained)
- 1 cup granulated sugar (divided)
- ½ cup unsalted butter (melted)
- 1 cup self-rising flour
- 1 cup milk
- 1 teaspoon vanilla extract (optional)
- ½ teaspoon ground cinnamon (optional)

Directions

1. **Preheat the Oven**: Preheat your oven to 350°F (175°C).
2. **Prepare the Peaches**: If using fresh peaches, peel and slice them. If using canned peaches, drain them well.
3. **Melt the Butter**: Pour the melted butter into a 9x13-inch baking dish.
4. **Mix the Batter**: In a bowl, combine 1 cup of sugar, self-rising flour, and milk. Add the vanilla extract if desired. Mix until just combined; the batter will be somewhat runny.
5. **Assemble the Cobbler**: Pour the batter over the melted butter in the baking dish. Do not stir. Then, layer the peaches on top of the batter. Sprinkle the remaining sugar and cinnamon over the peaches.
6. **Bake**: Bake in the preheated oven for 30-45 minutes, or until the top is golden brown and the cobbler is bubbling around the edges.
7. **Serve**: Allow to cool slightly before serving. Enjoy warm, ideally with a scoop of vanilla ice cream or whipped cream.

Cooking and Prep Time

- **Prep Time**: 15 minutes
- **Cooking Time**: 30-45 minutes

- **Total Time:** Approximately 1 hour

Nutrition Information (per serving)

- **Calories:** 250
- **Fat:** 10 g
- **Carbohydrates:** 38 g
- **Fiber:** 2 g
- **Sugar:** 20 g
- **Protein:** 3 g

8.10 Pineapple Upside-Down Cake

Ingredients

Topping:

- 1/2 cup (4 Tbsp; 56g) unsalted butter, melted
- 1/2 cup (100g) packed light or dark brown sugar
- 8–10 pineapple slices
- 15–20 maraschino cherries

Cake:

- 1 and 1/2 cups (177g) cake flour, spooned & leveled
- 1 teaspoon baking powder
- 1/4 teaspoon baking soda
- 1/2 teaspoon salt
- 6 Tablespoons (85g) unsalted butter, softened to room temperature
- 3/4 cup (150g) granulated sugar
- 2 large egg whites, at room temperature
- 1/3 cup (80g) sour cream, at room temperature
- 1 teaspoon pure vanilla extract
- 1/4 cup (60ml) pineapple juice, at room temperature (use leftover from can)
- 2 Tablespoons (30ml) milk, at room temperature

Directions

1. **Prepare the topping**: Melt the butter, pour into an un-greased cake pan or pie dish, sprinkle with brown sugar, then arrange the blotted pineapple rings and maraschino cherries.
2. **Prepare the cake batter**: Whisk the dry ingredients together. In a separate bowl, cream the butter and sugar together. Beat in the egg whites and vanilla, then the sour cream. Pour the dry into the wet ingredients, pour in the pineapple juice & milk, and then beat to combine.

3. **Spread over topping**: Pour and spread the cake batter over the chilled topping.
4. **Bake**: Because of the wet bottom layer (which is the topping), the cake takes much longer than a typical 1 layer cake. Its juices will bubble up the sides, creating these incredible caramelized edges.
5. **Cool**: Cool the cake for 20 minutes before inverting onto a serving plate. Inverting any sooner will create a seeping mess—we want the topping to "set" as much as it can.

Prep Time: 20 minutes

Cook Time: 55 minutes

Total Time: 1 hour 15 minutes

Serving: 8-10 servings

Nutritional Information for Pineapple Upside-Down Cake

The following nutritional values are based on a serving size of one piece (approximately 115g):

- **Calories**: 367
- **Total Fat**: 13.9g (18% DV)
    - Saturated Fat: 3.4g (17% DV)
    - Trans Fat: Not specified
- **Cholesterol**: 25.3mg (8% DV)
- **Sodium**: 366.8mg (15% DV)
- **Total Carbohydrate**: 58.1g (21% DV)
    - Dietary Fiber: 0.92g (3% DV)
    - Sugars: Not specified
- **Protein**: 4g (8% DV)

Vitamins and Minerals

- **Vitamin C**: 1.4mg (2% DV)
- **Calcium**: 138mg (11% DV)
- **Iron**: 1.7mg (9% DV)

- **Potassium**: 128.8mg (3% DV)
- **Phosphorus**: 94.3mg (8% DV)

8.11 Oatmeal Cookies

Ingredients

- **1 1/2 cups** old-fashioned oats
- **3/4 cup** all-purpose flour
- **1 teaspoon** ground cinnamon
- **3/4 teaspoon** fine sea salt
- **1/2 teaspoon** baking soda
- **1/2 cup** unsalted butter, room temperature
- **2/3 cup** packed light brown sugar
- **1 large egg**
- **1 teaspoon** vanilla extract
- **Optional add-ins**: up to 1 cup total (e.g., raisins, chocolate chips, chopped nuts)

Directions

1. **Combine Dry Ingredients**: In a medium bowl, mix together the oats, flour, cinnamon, salt, and baking soda.
2. **Mix Wet Ingredients**: In a large bowl, cream the softened butter and brown sugar until light and fluffy (about 2 minutes). Add the egg and vanilla extract, beating until combined.
3. **Combine Mixtures**: Gradually add the dry ingredients to the wet mixture, mixing on low speed until just combined.
4. **Add Optional Ingredients**: If desired, fold in any add-ins like chocolate chips or raisins.
5. **Chill the Dough**: Transfer the dough to a container and refrigerate for at least 1-2 hours to firm up.
6. **Preheat Oven**: Preheat your oven to 350°F (180°C) and line a baking sheet with parchment paper.

7. **Shape Cookies**: Use a medium cookie scoop to form balls of dough (about 2 tablespoons each) and place them on the prepared baking sheet, spacing them a few inches apart.
8. **Bake**: Bake for 10-12 minutes or until the cookies are lightly golden around the edges and the centers are set.
9. **Cool**: Let the cookies cool on the baking sheet for 5 minutes before transferring them to a wire rack to cool completely.

Cooking and Prep Time

- **Prep Time**: 20 minutes (plus chilling time)
- **Cook Time**: 10-12 minutes
- **Total Time**: Approximately 1 hour (including chilling)

Serving

- Makes about **24 cookies** (depending on size).

Nutritional Information (per cookie, based on 24 servings)

- **Calories**: 150
- **Total Fat**: 7g (11% DV)
    - Saturated Fat: 4g (20% DV)
- **Cholesterol**: 15mg (5% DV)
- **Sodium**: 75mg (3% DV)
- **Total Carbohydrates**: 20g (7% DV)
    - Dietary Fiber: 1g (4% DV)
    - Sugars: 8g
- **Protein**: 2g (4% DV)

Vitamins and Minerals

- **Calcium**: 10mg (1% DV)
- **Iron**: 0.5mg (3% DV)

8.12 Strawberry Shortcake

Ingredients

For the Biscuits:

- **2 and 3/4 cups** (345g) all-purpose flour
- **1/4 cup** (50g) granulated sugar
- **4 teaspoons** baking powder
- **1/2 teaspoon** baking soda
- **1 teaspoon** fine sea salt
- **3/4 cup** (170g) unsalted butter, cold and cubed
- **1 cup** (240ml) cold buttermilk

For the Strawberries:

- **6–7 cups** fresh strawberries, quartered
- **1/4 cup + 2 tablespoons** (75g) granulated sugar, divided
- **1 teaspoon** pure vanilla extract

For the Whipped Cream:

- **1 cup** (240ml) heavy cream
- **2 tablespoons** (30g) powdered sugar
- **1 teaspoon** pure vanilla extract

Directions

1. **Prepare the Strawberries**: In a bowl, combine the quartered strawberries with 1/4 cup of sugar and vanilla extract. Let them sit for at least 30 minutes to macerate, allowing the juices to develop.
2. **Make the Biscuits**: Preheat your oven to 425°F (220°C). In a large bowl, whisk together the flour, sugar, baking powder, baking soda, and salt. Cut in the cold butter using a pastry cutter or your fingers until the mixture resembles coarse crumbs. Stir in the buttermilk until just combined.

3. **Shape the Biscuits**: Turn the dough onto a floured surface and gently knead it a few times. Pat it into a rectangle about 1-inch thick. Cut out biscuits using a round cutter and place them on a baking sheet lined with parchment paper.
4. **Bake the Biscuits**: Bake for 12-15 minutes or until golden brown. Remove from the oven and let them cool slightly.
5. **Prepare the Whipped Cream**: In a mixing bowl, beat the heavy cream, powdered sugar, and vanilla extract until soft peaks form.
6. **Assemble the Shortcakes**: Slice the biscuits in half. Spoon a generous amount of the macerated strawberries over the bottom half, add a dollop of whipped cream, and then top with the other half of the biscuit. Serve immediately.

Cooking and Prep Time

- **Prep Time**: 30 minutes (plus macerating time)
- **Cook Time**: 15 minutes
- **Total Time**: Approximately 1 hour

Serving

- Makes about **8 servings**.

Nutritional Information (per serving)

- **Calories**: 320
- **Total Fat**: 18g (28% DV)
    - Saturated Fat: 10g (50% DV)
- **Cholesterol**: 60mg (20% DV)
- **Sodium**: 250mg (11% DV)
- **Total Carbohydrates**: 36g (12% DV)
    - Dietary Fiber: 1g (4% DV)
    - Sugars: 14g
- **Protein**: 4g (8% DV)

Vitamins and Minerals

- **Calcium**: 150mg (12% DV)

- **Iron**: 1mg (6% DV)

8.13 Almond Flour Brownies

Ingredients

For the Brownies:

- **1 1/2 cups** (180g) almond flour
- **3/4 cup** (64g) unsweetened cocoa powder
- **1 teaspoon** baking powder
- **1/2 teaspoon** salt
- **5 tablespoons** (70g) unsalted butter, melted
- **1 1/2 cups** (300g) granulated sugar (or sweetener of choice)
- **3 large eggs** (room temperature)
- **1 teaspoon** vanilla extract
- **1/2 cup** (85g) chocolate chips (optional)

Directions

1. **Preheat the Oven**: Preheat your oven to 350°F (177°C). Line an 8x8-inch baking pan with parchment paper, leaving some overhang for easy removal later.
2. **Mix Dry Ingredients**: In a medium bowl, whisk together the almond flour, cocoa powder, baking powder, and salt until well combined.
3. **Combine Wet Ingredients**: In a large bowl, whisk together the melted butter, granulated sugar, eggs, and vanilla extract until smooth and well combined.
4. **Combine Mixtures**: Gradually add the dry ingredients to the wet ingredients, mixing until just combined. If using, fold in the chocolate chips.
5. **Bake**: Pour the brownie batter into the prepared baking pan and spread it evenly. Bake for 33-38 minutes, or until a toothpick inserted into the center comes out clean or with a few moist crumbs.
6. **Cool**: Allow the brownies to cool in the pan for about 15-20 minutes before lifting them out using the parchment paper. Let them cool completely on a wire rack before slicing.

Cooking and Prep Time

- **Prep Time**: 10 minutes
- **Cook Time**: 35-38 minutes
- **Total Time**: Approximately 50-60 minutes

Serving

- Makes about **12 servings**.

Nutritional Information (per brownie, based on 12 servings)

- **Calories**: 200
- **Total Fat**: 12g (18% DV)
    - Saturated Fat: 7g (35% DV)
- **Cholesterol**: 50mg (17% DV)
- **Sodium**: 80mg (3% DV)
- **Total Carbohydrates**: 22g (8% DV)
    - Dietary Fiber: 3g (12% DV)
    - Sugars: 14g
- **Protein**: 4g (8% DV)

Vitamins and Minerals

- **Calcium**: 30mg (2% DV)
- **Iron**: 1.5mg (8% DV)

8.14 Carrot Cake

Ingredients

For the Cake:

- **2 ½ cups** (300g) all-purpose flour
- **2 teaspoons** baking powder
- **1 teaspoon** baking soda
- **1 teaspoon** salt
- **1 teaspoon** ground cinnamon
- **½ teaspoon** ground nutmeg
- **1⅓ cups** (320ml) vegetable oil
- **1 cup** (220g) packed light brown sugar
- **1 cup** (200g) granulated sugar
- **4 large eggs**
- **2 teaspoons** vanilla extract
- **3 cups** (315g) grated carrots (about 1 pound of carrots)
- **1 cup** (120g) chopped pecans (optional)

For the Cream Cheese Frosting:

- **1 (8-ounce)** (227g) block cream cheese, room temperature
- **1 cup** (227g) unsalted butter, softened
- **1 teaspoon** vanilla extract
- **4 to 5 cups** (480-600g) powdered sugar

Directions

1. **Preheat the Oven**: Preheat your oven to 350°F (180°C). Grease two 9-inch round cake pans and line the bottoms with parchment paper.
2. **Mix Dry Ingredients**: In a large bowl, whisk together the flour, baking powder, baking soda, salt, cinnamon, and nutmeg.

3. **Mix Wet Ingredients**: In another bowl, whisk together the vegetable oil, brown sugar, granulated sugar, eggs, and vanilla extract until well combined.
4. **Combine Mixtures**: Pour the wet mixture into the dry mixture and stir until just combined. Do not overmix. Fold in the grated carrots and chopped pecans, if using.
5. **Bake**: Divide the batter evenly between the prepared cake pans. Bake for 30 to 35 minutes, or until a toothpick inserted into the center comes out clean. Allow the cakes to cool in the pans for 10 minutes before transferring to a wire rack to cool completely.
6. **Prepare the Frosting**: In a mixing bowl, beat the cream cheese until smooth. Add the softened butter and mix until well combined. Gradually add powdered sugar and vanilla extract, mixing until fluffy and spreadable.
7. **Assemble the Cake**: Once the cake layers are completely cool, place one layer on a serving plate. Spread about ¾ cup of frosting over the top. Place the second layer on top and frost the top and sides of the cake with the remaining frosting. Decorate with additional chopped pecans if desired.

Cooking and Prep Time

- **Prep Time**: 30 minutes
- **Cook Time**: 30-35 minutes
- **Total Time**: Approximately 1 hour

Serving

- Makes about **12 servings**.

Nutritional Information (per serving)

- **Calories**: 410
- **Total Fat**: 25g (38% DV)
    - Saturated Fat: 10g (50% DV)
- **Cholesterol**: 80mg (27% DV)
- **Sodium**: 350mg (15% DV)
- **Total Carbohydrates**: 45g (15% DV)

    - Dietary Fiber: 2g (8% DV)
    - Sugars: 30g
- **Protein**: 4g (8% DV)

Vitamins and Minerals

- **Calcium**: 50mg (4% DV)
- **Iron**: 1.5mg (8% DV)

Chapter 8: Beverage Recipes

9.1 Herbal Teas

Ingredients for Basic Herbal Tea

- **1-2 teaspoons** dried herbs or 2-3 tablespoons fresh herbs
- **1 cup** boiling water

Directions

1. **Choose your herbs**: Select 1-2 teaspoons of dried herbs or 2-3 tablespoons of fresh herbs. Some popular options include:
- Peppermint
- Chamomile
- Ginger
- Lemon balm
- Rosemary
- Dandelion
- Hibiscus
- Lavender
2. **Place the herbs in a teapot or mug**: If using dried herbs, place them directly in the pot/mug. For fresh herbs, place them in an infuser or tea bag.
3. **Pour boiling water over the herbs**: Fill your pot or mug with 1 cup of freshly boiled water.
4. **Steep for 5-10 minutes**: Allow the tea to steep for 5-10 minutes, depending on the herb. The longer it steeps, the stronger the flavor will be.
5. **Strain and serve**: If using loose herbs, strain the tea into your cup. Add any desired sweeteners like honey or lemon.

Prep Time: 5 minutes

Cook Time: 5-10 minutes

Total Time: 10-15 minutes

Serving: 1 cup

Herbal teas are a delicious and healthy way to enjoy the benefits of herbs. They are naturally caffeine-free and can be enjoyed hot or iced. The nutritional value varies depending on the herbs used, but many provide antioxidants, vitamins, and minerals. Some potential health benefits of herbal teas include:

- Peppermint tea may aid digestion and relieve nausea
- Chamomile tea has anti-inflammatory properties and may promote relaxation
- Ginger tea may help reduce inflammation and nausea
- Dandelion tea is a natural diuretic and may support liver health

9.2 Infused Water

Ingredients for Infused Water

Basic Infused Water

- **1 liter** (about 4 cups) of water
- **1-2 cups** of fresh fruits, vegetables, or herbs (choose your favorites)

Popular Combinations

- **Citrus Infusion**:
    - 1 orange, sliced
    - 1 lemon, sliced
    - 1 lime, sliced
- **Berry Infusion**:
    - 1 cup mixed berries (strawberries, blueberries, raspberries)
- **Herbal Infusion**:
    - 1 cup fresh mint leaves
    - 1 cucumber, sliced
- **Tropical Infusion**:
    - 1 cup pineapple chunks
    - 1 lime, sliced

Directions

1. **Prepare Ingredients**: Wash and slice the fruits, vegetables, or herbs as needed. For herbs, you can gently bruise them to release more flavor.
2. **Combine in a Pitcher**: In a large pitcher, add your chosen fruits, vegetables, or herbs.
3. **Add Water**: Pour in 1 liter of water over the ingredients.
4. **Infuse**: Allow the mixture to infuse in the refrigerator for at least 1-2 hours. For stronger flavor, let it sit overnight.

5. **Serve**: Pour the infused water into glasses over ice if desired. You can also add additional slices of the fruits or herbs for garnish.

Prep Time: 10 minutes

Infusion Time: 1-12 hours (depending on desired strength)

Total Time: Approximately 10 minutes plus infusion time

Serving

- Makes about **4 servings** (1 liter).

Nutritional Information (per serving)

Infused water is generally low in calories and contains no fat, cholesterol, or significant carbohydrates. Here are some approximate values based on a basic fruit infusion:

- **Calories**: 5-10 (depending on the fruits used)
- **Total Fat**: 0g
- **Sodium**: 0mg
- **Total Carbohydrates**: 1-2g
    - Sugars: 1g
- **Protein**: 0g

Vitamins and Minerals

The nutritional content will vary based on the fruits and herbs used, but infused water can provide some vitamins and antioxidants from the ingredients. For example:

- Citrus fruits are high in Vitamin C.
- Berries are rich in antioxidants.
- Cucumbers are hydrating and low in calories.

9.3 Kidney-Friendly Smoothies

Ingredients

- **1 cup** plain, unsweetened plant milk (e.g., almond milk or cashew milk)
- **1/4 cup** unsweetened plant yogurt (optional)
- **1 tablespoon** ground flaxseed
- **1 tablespoon** chia seeds
- **1 cup** raw leafy greens (e.g., spinach or kale)
- **1 cup** frozen pineapple
- **1/2 cup** frozen blueberries (or a mixed berry blend)

Directions

1. **Prepare Ingredients**: Gather all ingredients. If using fresh leafy greens, wash them thoroughly.
2. **Layer Ingredients in Blender**: Start by adding the plant milk to the blender, followed by the plant yogurt (if using), ground flaxseed, chia seeds, leafy greens, and frozen fruits.
3. **Blend**: Blend on high until smooth and creamy. If the mixture is too thick, you can add a little more plant milk to reach your desired consistency.
4. **Taste and Adjust**: Taste the smoothie and adjust the sweetness if necessary. You can add a little honey or a sweetener of your choice, but keep in mind the dietary restrictions for kidney health.
5. **Serve**: Pour the smoothie into a glass and enjoy immediately. You can also store any leftovers in the fridge for up to 24 hours.

Cooking and Prep Time

- **Prep Time**: 10 minutes
- **Total Time**: 10 minutes

Serving

- Makes **1 serving**.

Nutritional Information (per smoothie)

- **Calories**: 301
- **Total Fat**: 9g (14% DV)
    - Saturated Fat: 1g (5% DV)
- **Cholesterol**: 0mg (0% DV)
- **Sodium**: 150mg (6% DV)
- **Total Carbohydrates**: 45g (15% DV)
    - Dietary Fiber: 12g (48% DV)
    - Sugars: 18g
- **Protein**: 7.5g (15% DV)
- **Potassium**: 513mg (15% DV)
- **Phosphorus**: 140mg (11% DV)

Vitamins and Minerals

- **Calcium**: Varies based on plant milk used
- **Iron**: Varies based on leafy greens used

9.4 Low-Sugar Lemonade

Ingredients for Low-Sugar Lemonade

- **3-4 fresh lemons** (or 1/2 cup lemon juice)
- **4 cups filtered water**
- **1/4 cup honey or maple syrup** (or more to taste)

Directions

1. **Make a simple syrup**: In a small saucepan, combine 1 cup of water with your sweetener of choice (honey or maple syrup) over medium heat. Stir occasionally until the sweetener is fully dissolved. Remove from heat and let cool slightly.
2. **Juice the lemons**: Juice 3-4 lemons to obtain 1/2 cup of fresh lemon juice. Strain the juice to remove pulp and seeds if desired.
3. **Combine ingredients**: In a pitcher, combine the lemon juice, remaining 3 cups of water, and the simple syrup. Stir well to mix.
4. **Chill and serve**: Refrigerate the lemonade until chilled, at least 30 minutes. Serve over ice and garnish with lemon slices if desired.

Prep Time: 10 minutes

Cook Time: 5 minutes

Total Time: 15 minutes

Serving: Makes about 4 servings (1 cup each)

Nutrition Information (per serving)

- **Calories**: 60
- **Total Fat**: 0g
- **Sodium**: 5mg
- **Total Carbohydrates**: 16g
    - Dietary Fiber: 0g
    - Sugars: 14g
- **Protein**: 0g

9.5 Green Juice

Ingredients

- 3 celery ribs, halved
- 1/2 medium cucumber, sliced
- 2 large kale leaves (or 5 oz baby spinach, or half a head of romaine lettuce)
- 1 medium sweet apple (such as Gala or Honeycrisp), cored and cut into chunks
- 3/4-inch knob of fresh ginger, peeled
- 1/2 large lime (or 1/2 small lemon), peeled

Directions

1. **Prepare Ingredients**: Wash all fruits and vegetables thoroughly. Cut the celery, cucumber, apple, and ginger into manageable pieces for your juicer.
2. **Juicing**: Add the prepared ingredients to an electric juicer in batches. Start with the softer ingredients like apple and cucumber to help push through the harder ones like celery and kale.
3. **Serve**: Once all ingredients are juiced, stir the juice to mix well. Serve immediately over ice or transfer to an airtight container and refrigerate for up to 24 hours.

Cooking and Prep Time

- **Prep Time**: 5 minutes
- **Juicing Time**: 5 minutes
- **Total Time**: 10 minutes

Serving

- Makes about **2 cups** (2 servings).

Nutritional Information (per serving)

- **Calories**: 80
- **Total Fat**: 1g (2% DV)
- **Sodium**: 15mg (1% DV)

- **Total Carbohydrates**: 20g (7% DV)
    - Dietary Fiber: 3g (12% DV)
    - Sugars: 12g
- **Protein**: 2g (4% DV)

Vitamins and Minerals

- **Vitamin A**: 3355 IU (67% DV)
- **Vitamin C**: 46.4 mg (56% DV)
- **Calcium**: 65 mg (7% DV)
- **Iron**: 0.8 mg (4% DV)
- **Potassium**: 374 mg (11% DV)

9.6 Iced Tea

Ingredients for Iced Tea

- **8 tea bags** (black tea, green tea, or herbal tea)
- **1/2 cup** boiling water
- **7 1/2 cups** cold water
- **1/4 cup** sugar or honey (optional)
- **1 lemon**, sliced (optional garnish)

Directions

1. **Steep the tea**: Place the tea bags in a heat-proof pitcher. Pour the boiling water over the tea bags and let steep for 5-7 minutes. Remove the tea bags.
2. **Sweeten (optional)**: If desired, stir in the sugar or honey until dissolved. The amount of sweetener can be adjusted to taste.
3. **Dilute with cold water**: Add the cold water to the tea concentrate. Stir to combine.
4. **Chill**: Refrigerate the iced tea for at least 2 hours or until completely chilled.
5. **Serve**: Pour the iced tea over ice in glasses. Garnish with lemon slices if desired.

Prep Time: 5 minutes

Cook Time: 5-7 minutes (steeping)

Total Time: 2 hours 10 minutes (including chilling)

Serving: Makes about 8 servings (1 cup each)

Nutritional Information (per serving)

- **Calories**: 43
- **Total Fat**: 0g
- **Sodium**: 24mg (1% DV)
- **Total Carbohydrates**: 12g (4% DV)
  - Dietary Fiber: 0g
  - Sugars: 12g (13% DV)

- **Protein**: 1g (2% DV)

Vitamins and Minerals

- **Calcium**: 14mg (1% DV)
- **Iron**: 1mg (6% DV)

9.7 Coconut Water

beverage that provides essential electrolytes and nutrients. Here are the key nutrition facts for a typical 8-ounce (240 ml) serving of coconut water:

- **Calories**: 45-60
- **Total Fat**: 0g
- **Cholesterol**: 0mg
- **Sodium**: 25-252mg
- **Potassium**: 470-600mg
- **Total Carbohydrates**: 9-11g
- **Sugars**: 6-11g
- **Protein**: 0.5-2g
- **Vitamin C**: 10% DV
- **Calcium**: 4-6% DV
- **Magnesium**: 4-15% DV

Coconut water is an excellent source of potassium, providing about 15% of the recommended daily intake in a single cup. It also contains small amounts of other essential minerals like calcium, magnesium, and phosphorus.

Health Benefits

Coconut water offers several potential health benefits:

1. **Provides electrolytes and aids in hydration**, making it a good choice for post-workout recovery
2. **May help reduce blood pressure and stroke risk** due to its high potassium content
3. **Contains antioxidants** that may help neutralize oxidative stress
4. **May promote kidney health** by helping to prevent kidney stones
5. **May have a moisturizing effect** on skin and help reduce signs of aging

Serving and Preparation

Coconut water can be enjoyed on its own, chilled, or used as a base for smoothies and other recipes. It requires no preparation other than refrigeration.

Coconut water is best consumed fresh, but it can be stored in the refrigerator for up to 5 days after opening.

9.8 Almond Milk Shake

Ingredients

- **1 cup** almond milk (unsweetened or vanilla)
- **1/2 banana** (optional for sweetness and creaminess)
- **1 tablespoon** agave nectar or honey (adjust to taste)
- **1 tablespoon** unsweetened cocoa powder (optional for chocolate flavor)
- **4-5 ice cubes**
- **1 scoop** protein powder (optional for added protein)

Directions

1. **Prepare Ingredients**: Gather all the ingredients. If using a banana, peel and slice it.
2. **Blend**: In a blender, combine the almond milk, banana, agave nectar (or honey), cocoa powder (if using), and ice cubes. If you want to add protein powder, include it as well.
3. **Blend Until Smooth**: Blend on high speed until the mixture is smooth and creamy. If you prefer a thicker shake, you can add more ice cubes and blend again.
4. **Taste and Adjust**: Taste the shake and adjust the sweetness if necessary by adding more agave nectar or honey.
5. **Serve**: Pour the almond milk shake into a glass and enjoy immediately. You can also garnish with a sprinkle of cocoa powder or a slice of banana on top if desired.

Cooking and Prep Time

- **Prep Time**: 5 minutes
- **Total Time**: 5 minutes

Serving

- Makes **1 serving** (approximately 12 ounces).

Nutritional Information (per serving)

- **Calories**: 200
- **Total Fat**: 5g (8% DV)
    - Saturated Fat: 0g (0% DV)
- **Cholesterol**: 0mg (0% DV)
- **Sodium**: 150mg (6% DV)
- **Total Carbohydrates**: 30g (10% DV)
    - Dietary Fiber: 4g (16% DV)
    - Sugars: 15g
- **Protein**: 5g (10% DV)

Vitamins and Minerals

- **Calcium**: 300mg (30% DV)
- **Iron**: 1mg (6% DV)
- **Potassium**: 400mg (11% DV)

9.9 Berry Blast Smoothie

Ingredients

- **1 banana**, preferably frozen
- **1 cup** frozen strawberries
- **1 cup** frozen blackberries
- **1 cup** frozen raspberries
- **1 1/4 cups** almond milk (or any milk of choice)
- **1/2 cup** Greek yogurt (optional for creaminess)
- **1 tablespoon** honey or agave nectar (optional, adjust to taste)

Directions

1. **Prepare Ingredients**: If you haven't done so, freeze the banana beforehand. Gather all the ingredients.
2. **Blend**: In a blender, combine the banana, frozen strawberries, blackberries, raspberries, almond milk, and Greek yogurt (if using).
3. **Sweeten (Optional)**: Add honey or agave nectar if you prefer a sweeter smoothie.
4. **Blend Until Smooth**: Blend on high until the mixture is smooth and creamy. If the smoothie is too thick, you can add a little more almond milk to achieve your desired consistency.
5. **Serve**: Pour the smoothie into a glass and enjoy immediately. You can also garnish with a few fresh berries or a slice of banana on top if desired.

Cooking and Prep Time

- **Prep Time**: 5 minutes
- **Total Time**: 5 minutes

Serving

- Makes about **2 servings** (approximately 16 ounces total).

Nutritional Information (per serving)

- **Calories**: 230
- **Total Fat**: 3g (5% DV)
  - Saturated Fat: 1g (5% DV)
- **Cholesterol**: 5mg (2% DV)
- **Sodium**: 80mg (3% DV)
- **Total Carbohydrates**: 45g (15% DV)
  - Dietary Fiber: 6g (24% DV)
  - Sugars: 25g
- **Protein**: 8g (16% DV)

Vitamins and Minerals

- **Vitamin C**: 40% DV
- **Calcium**: 15% DV
- **Iron**: 4% DV
- **Potassium**: 10% DV

9.10 Ginger Tea

Ingredients

- **1 ½ teaspoons** freshly grated ginger root
- **1 ½ cups** boiling water
- **1-2 teaspoons** sugar or honey (optional, to taste)
- **Lemon slice** (optional, for garnish)

Directions

1. **Prepare the Ginger**: Grate the fresh ginger root using a fine grater or a microplane.
2. **Steep the Ginger**: Place the grated ginger into a heatproof measuring cup or a teapot. Pour the boiling water over the ginger.
3. **Set Timer**: Allow the ginger to steep for about 10 minutes. This will extract the flavor and health benefits from the ginger.
4. **Strain the Tea**: After steeping, strain the tea into a mug to remove the ginger pieces.
5. **Sweeten (Optional)**: Stir in sugar or honey to taste, if desired. You can also add a squeeze of lemon for extra flavor.
6. **Serve**: Enjoy your ginger tea hot, or let it cool and serve over ice for a refreshing iced version.

Cooking and Prep Time

- **Prep Time**: 5 minutes
- **Steeping Time**: 10 minutes
- **Total Time**: 15 minutes

Serving

- Makes **1 serving**.

Nutritional Information (per serving)

- **Calories**: 30 (without added sweetener)
- **Total Fat**: 0g
- **Sodium**: 0mg
- **Total Carbohydrates**: 8g
    - Sugars: 8g (if sweetened)
- **Protein**: 0g

Vitamins and Minerals

- **Vitamin C**: 1% DV (from lemon, if added)
- **Potassium**: Approximately 40mg

9.11 Cucumber Mint Water

Ingredients

- **1 medium cucumber**, sliced
- **1/2 cup** fresh mint leaves
- **8 cups** filtered water
- **Ice cubes** (optional)

Directions

1. **Prepare Ingredients**: Wash the cucumber and mint leaves thoroughly. Slice the cucumber into thin rounds.
2. **Combine in a Pitcher**: In a large pitcher, add the sliced cucumber and fresh mint leaves.
3. **Add Water**: Pour the filtered water over the cucumber and mint.
4. **Infuse**: Allow the mixture to sit in the refrigerator for at least 1-2 hours to let the flavors infuse. For a stronger flavor, you can let it infuse overnight.
5. **Serve**: Pour the cucumber mint water into glasses over ice if desired. Garnish with additional cucumber slices or mint leaves for presentation.

Cooking and Prep Time

- **Prep Time**: 10 minutes
- **Infusion Time**: 1-12 hours (depending on desired strength)
- **Total Time**: Approximately 10 minutes plus infusion time

Serving

- Makes about **8 servings** (1 cup each).

Nutritional Information (per serving)

- **Calories**: 5
- **Total Fat**: 0g
- **Sodium**: 0mg

- **Total Carbohydrates**: 1g
    - Sugars: 0g
- **Protein**: 0g

Vitamins and Minerals

- **Vitamin C**: Minimal amounts from mint
- **Potassium**: Approximately 50mg from cucumber

9.12 Apple Cinnamon Water

Ingredients

- 1 medium apple, sliced
- 2-3 cinnamon sticks
- 8 cups filtered water
- Ice cubes (optional)

Directions

1. **Prepare Ingredients**: Wash the apple thoroughly. Cut it into thin slices, leaving the skin on for color and extra nutrients.
2. **Combine in a Pitcher**: In a large pitcher, add the apple slices and cinnamon sticks.
3. **Add Water**: Pour the filtered water over the apple and cinnamon.
4. **Infuse**: Allow the mixture to sit in the refrigerator for at least 2-3 hours to let the flavors infuse. For a stronger flavor, you can let it infuse overnight.
5. **Serve**: Remove the cinnamon sticks. Pour the apple cinnamon water into glasses over ice if desired. Garnish with additional apple slices for presentation.

Prep Time

- **Prep Time**: 10 minutes
- **Infusion Time**: 2-12 hours (depending on desired strength)
- **Total Time**: Approximately 10 minutes plus infusion time

Serving

- Makes about **8 servings** (1 cup each).

Nutritional Information (per serving)

- **Calories**: 10
- **Total Fat**: 0g
- **Sodium**: 0mg

- **Total Carbohydrates**: 2g
    - Dietary Fiber: 0g
    - Sugars: 1g
- **Protein**: 0g

Vitamins and Minerals

- **Vitamin C**: 1% DV
- **Potassium**: 30mg

9.13 Chamomile Tea

Ingredients

- 1-2 teaspoons dried chamomile flowers or 1 chamomile tea bag
- 1 cup boiling water
- 1 teaspoon honey or sugar (optional, to taste)
- Lemon slice (optional, for garnish)

Directions

1. **Prepare the Chamomile**: If using dried chamomile flowers, measure out 1-2 teaspoons. If using a tea bag, simply have it ready.
2. **Boil Water**: Bring water to a rolling boil.
3. **Steep the Tea**: In a cup or teapot, add the chamomile flowers or tea bag. Pour the boiling water over the chamomile and let it steep for about 5 minutes.
4. **Sweeten (Optional)**: If desired, stir in honey or sugar to taste.
5. **Serve**: Remove the tea bag or strain out the chamomile flowers. Garnish with a lemon slice if desired. Enjoy your chamomile tea hot, or let it cool and serve over ice for a refreshing iced version.

Prep Time

- **Prep Time**: 5 minutes
- **Steeping Time**: 5 minutes
- **Total Time**: 10 minutes

Serving

- Makes **1 serving**.

Nutritional Information (per serving)

- **Calories**: 2 (without added sweetener)
- **Total Fat**: 0g
- **Sodium**: 0mg

- **Total Carbohydrates**: 1g
  - Sugars: 0g
- **Protein**: 0g

Vitamins and Minerals

- **Calcium**: Minimal amounts
- **Iron**: Minimal amounts

9.14 Turmeric Latte

Ingredients

- 1-2 cups milk of choice (dairy, almond, coconut, etc.)
- 1-2 teaspoons ground turmeric
- ¼ teaspoon ground cinnamon
- ¼ teaspoon ground ginger or 1/2 inch fresh grated ginger
- Pinch of black pepper
- 1 teaspoon honey or maple syrup (optional)
- Vanilla extract (optional)

Directions

1. In a saucepan, whisk together the milk, turmeric, cinnamon, ginger, and black pepper.
2. Heat the mixture over medium heat, whisking frequently, until steaming and hot but not boiling.
3. Remove from heat and stir in honey or maple syrup if using.
4. Pour the turmeric latte through a fine mesh strainer into mugs.
5. Top with a sprinkle of cinnamon or froth the milk using a milk frother or blender for a foamy texture.

Prep and Cook Time

- **Prep time**: 2-5 minutes
- **Cook time**: 5-10 minutes
- **Total time**: 7-15 minutes

Serving

This recipe makes 1-2 servings of turmeric latte, depending on the amount of milk used.

Nutrition (per serving)

- **Calories**: 48-96 kcal
- **Carbohydrates**: 4-8g

- **Protein**: 1-2g
- **Fat**: 2-4g

Turmeric provides anti-inflammatory and antioxidant benefits from the compound curcumin.

Chapter 9: Special Diets and Adjustments

10.1 Vegetarian and Vegan Options

Incorporating vegetarian and vegan options into your diet can be beneficial for managing Stage 3 kidney disease. Plant-based diets often emphasize nutrient-dense foods that can help manage kidney health by reducing the intake of animal proteins and potentially lowering phosphorus levels. Here are some tips for including vegetarian and vegan options in your diet:

- **Protein Sources:** Opt for plant-based proteins like tofu, tempeh, lentils, and chickpeas. These can be lower in phosphorus and can be a great alternative to animal proteins.
- **Low-Potassium Vegetables:** Choose vegetables like bell peppers, cabbage, carrots, and cauliflower. These can be steamed, sautéed, or added to salads and casseroles.
- **Grains:** Include refined grains like white rice, pasta, and white bread. These grains typically have lower phosphorus content compared to whole grains.
- **Dairy Alternatives:** Use unsweetened almond milk or rice milk as substitutes for dairy milk. These options are often lower in potassium and phosphorus.
- **Snacks:** Snack on unsalted rice cakes, fresh fruit, or vegetable sticks with hummus. These provide nutrients without excessive sodium or phosphorus.

By incorporating these plant-based options, you can create a kidney-friendly vegetarian or vegan diet that supports your health and nutritional needs.

10.2 Adjusting Recipes for Diabetic Patients

Adjusting recipes for diabetic patients with Stage 3 kidney disease requires careful consideration to manage both blood sugar levels and kidney health. Here are some tips for making kidney-friendly recipes suitable for diabetic patients:

- **Carbohydrate Control:** Choose complex carbohydrates with a low glycemic index, such as whole grains, legumes, and non-starchy vegetables. Monitor portion sizes to manage blood sugar levels.
- **Healthy Proteins:** Incorporate lean proteins like chicken, turkey, fish, tofu, and legumes. Avoid high-fat and processed meats.
- **Low-Sodium Ingredients:** Use herbs, spices, and salt-free seasonings to enhance flavor without adding sodium. Opt for low-sodium versions of canned goods and broths.
- **Healthy Fats:** Include sources of healthy fats, such as olive oil, avocados, and nuts (in moderation, considering phosphorus content).
- **Sugar Substitutes:** Use sugar substitutes like stevia or erythritol in place of sugar to reduce the impact on blood glucose levels.
- **Monitor Potassium and Phosphorus:** Choose low-potassium fruits and vegetables, and be mindful of phosphorus content in foods.

By making these adjustments, you can create recipes that are both kidney-friendly and suitable for managing diabetes.

Chapter 10: Managing Dietary Challenges

11.1 Overcoming Appetite Loss

Appetite loss is common in patients with Stage 3 kidney disease, but it's important to maintain adequate nutrition. Here are some tips to overcome appetite loss:

- **Small, Frequent Meals:** Eat smaller portions more frequently throughout the day to make eating less overwhelming.
- **Nutrient-Dense Foods:** Choose high-calorie, nutrient-dense foods like nuts, seeds, avocados, and lean proteins to maximize nutrition with smaller amounts.
- **Appealing Foods:** Focus on foods that you enjoy and are visually appealing. Experiment with different textures, colors, and flavors to stimulate your appetite.
- **Meal Timing:** Eat your largest meal at the time of day when you feel most hungry, and take advantage of periods when your appetite is better.
- **Supplements:** Consider nutrient supplements or high-calorie drinks, but consult with your healthcare provider or dietitian to ensure they are appropriate for your dietary needs.

By following these strategies, you can better manage appetite loss and ensure you're getting the necessary nutrients to support your health.

11.2 Managing Nausea and Vomiting

Nausea and vomiting can be challenging for patients with Stage 3 kidney disease, but certain strategies can help manage these symptoms:

- **Eat Small, Frequent Meals:** Smaller, more frequent meals can be easier to tolerate and help prevent nausea.
- **Avoid Strong Smells:** Choose foods with mild odors and avoid cooking methods that produce strong smells, such as frying.
- **Stay Hydrated:** Sip clear fluids like water or herbal tea throughout the day to stay hydrated and ease nausea.
- **Ginger and Peppermint:** Ginger tea or peppermint candies can help soothe the stomach and reduce nausea.
- **Rest After Eating:** Sit upright or slightly reclined after eating to aid digestion and prevent vomiting.

By incorporating these tips, you can better manage nausea and vomiting and maintain your nutritional intake.

11.3 Dealing with Dietary Restrictions

Managing dietary restrictions in Stage 3 kidney disease can be challenging, but with the right approach, it becomes more manageable:

- **Understand Your Restrictions:** Learn about which foods to limit or avoid, such as those high in sodium, potassium, and phosphorus.
- **Focus on What You Can Eat:** Emphasize the wide variety of kidney-friendly foods available, such as certain fruits, vegetables, lean proteins, and refined grains.
- **Meal Planning:** Plan meals in advance to ensure they meet your dietary guidelines and provide balanced nutrition.
- **Creative Cooking:** Experiment with herbs, spices, and new recipes to make meals flavorful and enjoyable without added salt or high-phosphorus ingredients.
- **Seek Support:** Consult with a renal dietitian for personalized advice and support in navigating dietary restrictions effectively.

By focusing on these strategies, you can manage dietary restrictions while still enjoying satisfying and nutritious meals.

www.ingramcontent.com/pod-product-compliance
Lightning Source LLC
Chambersburg PA
CBHW082233220526
45479CB00005B/1214